D1141633

# Managing in Health and Social Care

## Essential checklists for frontline staff

William Bryans

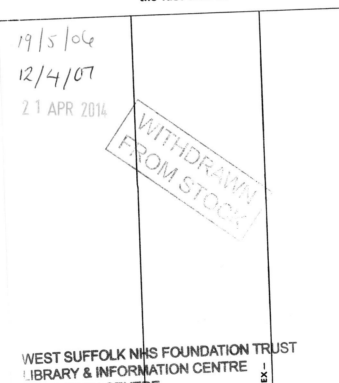
Radcliffe Medical Press

**Radcliffe Medical Press Ltd**
18 Marcham Road
Abingdon
Oxon OX14 1AA
United Kingdom

**www.radcliffe-oxford.com**
The Radcliffe Medical Press electronic catalogue and online ordering facility.
Direct sales to anywhere in the world.

---

British Library Cataloguing in Publication Data

A catalogue record for this book is available from the British Library.

ISBN 1 85775 856 0

Typeset by Aarontype Ltd, Easton, Bristol
Printed and bound by TJ International Ltd, Padstow, Cornwall

# Contents

About the author     iv

About this book     v

1   Promoting the culture of business competence     1

2   Gifts and hospitality     15

3   Cash and security matters     25

4   Planning essentials     37

5   Influencing the supply chain     53

6   Making a bid for additional resources     69

7   Making the most of budget management systems     79

8   Administration matters     93

Index     101

# About the author

**William Bryans** is a specialist in health and social services business and financial management. The material in this book is based upon his wide managerial experience, his involvement with organisation and management development (including the implementation of the Management Education System through Open Learning (MESOL) project, developed by the Institute of Healthcare Management as a mode of entry to the profession), and various published articles and papers.

As a promoter of the workplace as a management college, as a university lecturer and as an external assessor he has always been acutely aware of the need for definitive literature which brings together practical business advice. As well as providing checklists of actions to take in specific circumstances, this book gives definitions, guidance, facts and advice about complex matters in clear unambiguous language. It also provides a framework that can be adapted to meet individual needs.

William is a Fellow of the Chartered Institute of Secretaries and Administrators (FCIS) and a Fellow of the Institute of Healthcare Management (FHM).

# About this book

*Managing in Health and Social Care* focuses on the frequent occasions when frontline staff find themselves confronted for the first time by urgent problems associated with finance, legal or other administrative matters and are unsure how to proceed.

The checklists in this book provide a framework within which the performance of frontline staff who are confronted with unfamiliar business-type problems can be improved so that they:

- do the right thing
- at the right time
- every time.

In this context, frontline staff are defined as those who have little or no experience and/or limited knowledge of a business-oriented task that they have to undertake for the first time. Examples might include a ward sister or non-administrative departmental head having to organise a meeting, nurses or even paymaster staff having to deal with money matters or order communications (mechanised system for obtaining supplies, drugs, etc.), and so on.

Inexperience, negligence, inaccessible advice or ignorance of sound guidance can lead to all kinds of serious problems, including the potential for fraud, ineffectiveness and resource waste. This can be described as failure in the management process (*see* Figure A).

Process failure results in time and effort being wasted on correcting errors and making endless adjustments to take account of an escalating list of mistakes. It causes frustration and loss of motivation as well as opportunities for fraud, through what is perceived to be management ineffectiveness. Poor industrial relations can also be a consequence.

The essential checklists in this book improve the quality of the process by helping managers and staff to:

- do the right thing
- at the right time
- every time.

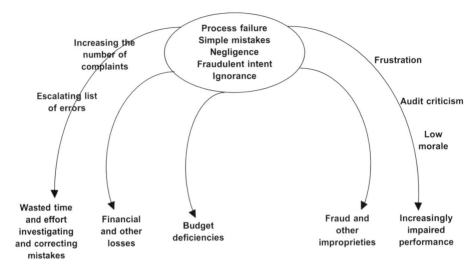

**Figure A**   Process failure cascade.

Although every authority and trust has its own regulations, often these are not immediately available to the hard-pressed ward sister, staff nurse, night staff or any of a multitude of other staff. Indeed, it is impossible to keep the thousands of staff on an acute hospital site properly briefed. However, the guidance and tips contained in this book do not contradict any internal rule or regulation, because they are based on sound simple business sense, and they will greatly enhance competence, confidence and effectiveness. The emphasis is on a 'what to do next' approach to unknown territory.

These essential checklists provide practical help and guidance in a readily accessible format. They will also help managers and other staff to review or rewrite business protocols.

## Aims of the book

This book sets out clearly and concisely how to tackle a variety of different problems in an accessible way, and cross-referencing is included where appropriate. The material is organised in such a way as to help managers and other frontline staff to:

- cope in work areas where they have little experience (e.g. handling gifts and cash)
- gain ready access to a wide spectrum of advice (e.g. influencing supply chain management)
- obtain guidance at critical moments (e.g. improving departmental relationships with the paymaster)

- improve their business, administrative and budget competence
- participate positively in a variety of processes (e.g. planning and organising a meeting)
- assemble coherent cases for additional resources
- help to improve existing conditions
- maintain a comprehensive source of reference.

## Who will benefit from this book?

Frontline staff are intended to be the main beneficiaries. This includes any member of staff who is obliged for the first time, or else only rarely, to undertake a business task of which they have little or no experience.

In addition to frontline staff, there is a significant shortage of published material that bridges the gap between principles and practice, and which is readily accessible to the prospective, first-time or mature manager who wants to check something out, update their own rules, write a protocol, or 'dip into' a particular business aspect. Although the book will be useful to a much wider readership, there is also a demand at postgraduate level both on the part of tutors who wish to update their knowledge and on the part of students who need to develop their competence in this complex area. This book will be of interest to all management levels, and will be an accessible handbook for those who wish to review current arrangements or design a fresh approach to practical business, administrative or financial problems. It should also provide up-to-date information and guidance for those engaged in general management.

## Promoting the culture of competence

- The material is firmly rooted in an ethos of securing process quality.
- Its application will therefore reduce mistakes and improve resource management by guiding staff to do the right thing, first time, every time.
- Readers will be assisted in tackling practical administrative and financial problems in a systematic and purposeful manner.
- It will be a guide to organisations, and will be useful to managers in all disciplines who are endeavouring to improve both their own performance and that of their services.
- Application of the principles described here will result in real savings in terms of staff occupied in the correction process.
- There will be improved morale and a reversal of feelings of despondency, leading to higher levels of competence and confidence.

- There will be an improved working environment and internal co-operation.
- There will be lower staff turnover, sickness levels and general absenteeism.
- There will be an enhanced capacity for internal scrutiny and the potential for further quality improvements.
- There will be greater respect from the workforce.

# Structure

The book contains around 30 checklists, each of which has a short supporting section that contains the following:

- a purpose statement and key-point analysis
- examples and diagrams, if appropriate
- hints for managers who wish to write a business protocol
- a checklist of practical steps for frontline staff who are confronted with the problem under consideration
- tips from the top
- part of an ongoing, semi-humorous case study that illustrates relevant aspects.

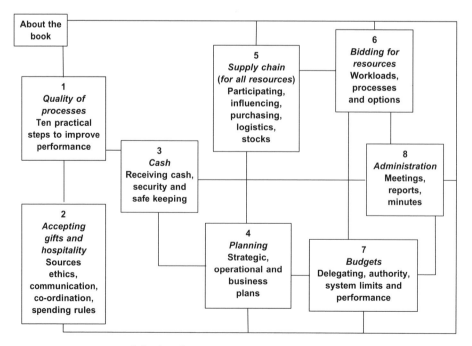

**Figure B**   Structure of the book.

As well as the lists of actions to be taken in specific circumstances, the book provides definitions, guidance, facts and advice about complex matters in clear unambiguous language. It also provides a framework that can be adapted to meet individual needs.

## Disclaimer

Whilst the case studies are based on real situations, all the details, names, etc. are pure fiction. Any similarity to persons or places is completely coincidental.

To Edith

# 1

# Promoting the culture of business competence

This chapter provides a framework within which the performance of front-line staff who are confronted with unfamiliar business-type problems can be improved so that they:

- do the right thing
- at the right time
- every time.

In this context, frontline staff are defined as those who have little or no experience and/or limited knowledge of a business-oriented task that they have to undertake for the first time. Examples might include a ward sister or non-administrative departmental head having to organise a meeting, nurses or even paymaster staff having to deal with money matters, order communications, and so on.

After reading this chapter you will:

- have a grasp of how the relationships between departments influence the efficiency and effectiveness of the business machine
- understand how the application of process quality management can improve performance and release resources for care and treatment
- have a working knowledge of project management in general, and how it can be applied to improve process quality in the business machine.

## The issues

Working within their own disciplines, all health and social care staff are expected to operate prime quality processes. However, the efficiency and effectiveness of administrative and financial systems are also strongly dependent on the competence of these staff, whose main priority, in the case of clinical or social disciplines, is focused on their patients and clients. Business matters are areas in which many frontline staff do not necessarily have expertise or experience.

Although these areas are not life-threatening in the way that clinical areas can be, serious consequences may result from simple mistakes, negligence or ignorance. Measured in terms of both morale and money, these have a debilitating effect on the organisation and cover a wide spectrum, including complaints, claims for negligence or non-compliance with contractual obligations, time and effort wasted in correcting errors, losses (financial and other), increased costs, budget deficits, fraud and other improprieties, impaired performance, audit criticism, frustration and low morale.

As was pointed out in the introduction, mistakes, negligence and fraud have wasteful repercussions that reduce the amount of money and time that can be devoted to the patient or client. Thus it makes sense to perform business tasks correctly so that the bureaucracy works smoothly and at a minimum cost. Below is a checklist of the benefits that can be derived from adequate processes.

---

**Checklist of process quality benefits**

▼ Reduced waste in terms of time, effort and money, and lower level of physical losses
▼ Budget savings reflected in increased resource capacity and the ability to handle more patients/clients
▼ Lower overall costs, with commensurate collateral advantages
▼ Increased confidence and competence
▼ Improved reputation and more secure market connection
▼ Higher levels of satisfaction and increased numbers, with the capacity to deal with them
▼ Reduced sickness, absenteeism, staff turnover, etc.

---

# Process quality as a central theme

The application of the principles of process quality will generate savings in terms of time, money and effort. Figure 1.1 provides an overview of the way in which the correct action generates the expected benefits.

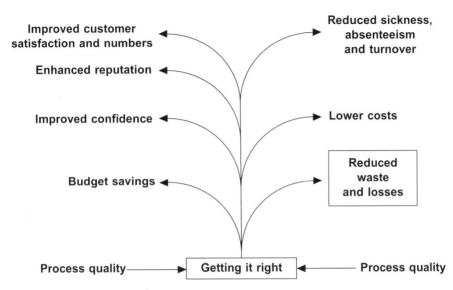

**Figure 1.1** Process quality in action.

This book explores the problems inherent in basic financial and administrative systems and shows how process quality can be improved. It aims to:

- assist frontline staff from all disciplines, including finance and administration, in tackling some of these problems with confidence
- improve overall process quality and performance
- reduce waste and cost
- help to maintain an efficient business machine that is facilitating rather than frustrating.

> Timing, meeting of appropriate deadlines, competence and communications are the main factors that influence process quality.

# Basic bureaucracy

The business systems that will be considered in this book have three main primary facets.

1  *Money coming into the system* (dealt with in sections devoted to cash receipts, gifts, etc.). Despite increasing reliance on other forms of payment, there is still a significant amount of cash in circulation (e.g. in dining rooms,

telephone boxes, vending machines, bank outlets, token machines, shops and other trading activities, and at ward level, patient/client monies, etc.).

The convenient transportability of money, particularly cash, makes it a high risk for fraud and theft. This means that rules are in place to protect the staff member, the organisation, and the person who is handing over the money. In addition, problems can arise from misdirection – for example:

- when money is received to settle an outstanding debt, but there is a failure to cancel the debt in the books of account, *or*
- where a gift is given for one purpose but is mistakenly used for another.

2   *Money being paid out* (i.e. expenditure, dealt with in sections devoted to influencing the supply chain, and payroll and personnel). This is a notoriously difficult area because there are so many links in the chain. At the very minimum these might include the following:

- the user who requires the goods or services
- the budget manager who gives authority
- the agent who supplies and personnel who initiate the purchase or recruit the member of staff through the issue of an order or contract
- the supplier or recruits who will indicate compliance or otherwise with the terms of the agreement
- the user who indicates receipt of goods and services or the arrival of the staff member in accordance with the agreed procedure
- the paymaster who pays for the goods and services or maintains the payroll.

3   *Administrative procedures involving, for example, planning, bidding for resources, organisation and management of meetings.* Skill and competence in these areas are important assets for the prospective and actual manager.

- The involvement of frontline staff may seem remote but often, in contrast to the paper-busy manager, they are in the best position to observe the reality of a situation and their views and opinions should therefore be sought.
- Comprehension of and participation in the planning cycle range from the strategic to implementation, and are in turn closely linked to bidding for resources and to budget management.
- The organisation and management of meetings are competences that are also related to process quality, for if there is insufficient preparation for a meeting (including one-to-one meetings between colleagues or between a senior and a junior member) then maximum and mutual benefit is unlikely to result.
- Where planning, budget management, etc. are on the agenda, these deficits become critical.

# The essential resources that money can buy

The spending of money (expenditure) obtains a wide spectrum of resources which, on a large hospital site, may be equivalent to the total requirements of a small town. These resources can be briefly categorised as shown in the following checklist.

---

**Checklist of resource categories**

▼   *Goods and services*: this includes a wide range of non-payroll spending, from direct clinical requirements to housekeeping and metered charges for telephones, water, heat, power and light.

▼   *Expertise*: directly employed staff (in hospitals this represents between 70% and 75% of the total running cost), and indirectly purchased personnel, such as independent contractors and agency staff.

▼   *Equipment*: all machines and electrical devices other than computers (see below) that are considered to be independent of the building fabric. There are a few exceptions. For example, an X-ray machine can be described as being both fixed and independent, but for this purpose it is regarded as equipment.

▼   *Systems*: this generally refers to information technology, and its effective use can be a worthwhile asset.

▼   *Estate*: this includes the building envelope, grounds, roadways, car parks, etc. together with the electrical and engineering infrastructure that supports tasks being undertaken.

---

As they are the prime users, whose actions initiate and sustain the supply lines, frontline and other staff have a major role to play in the management of these resources. This level of management does not require any sophisticated budgetary system. However, it does need a continual awareness of the implications for the process.

For example:

● use of the exact description or specification for the type of personnel, drugs or other clinical needs, goods, services, equipment, repairs, etc. that is required
● the correct manager to whom orders should be sent
● what to do when staff, goods, services or equipment:
  – do not arrive
  – are only part delivered
  – are damaged, faulty or in some way unsatisfactory

- how to commission resources
- how to stock, store and secure equipment and materials as well as drugs
- what to do when a stock of resources becomes redundant
- what to do when parts of the estate fall into disuse.

In addition to this list, there are many other areas where the correct action can save money, time and effort. Good stewardship enhances the individual's ability to participate in and contribute to planning and bidding for resources. The relationships are illustrated in Figure 1.2.

Improvement in process quality is best achieved through the positive participation on a multidisciplinary basis of all those who are involved in a chain of business-type transactions (e.g. heads of user departments, financial/paymaster managers, personnel/human resources, supply chain managers, etc.).

Managers have to evaluate and examine procedures, systems, structures and timing with a view to:

- creating a mutual understanding of all aspects of the supply/personnel/ paymaster problems
- identifying areas for improvement, particularly in the context of timing
- integrating systems and developing procedures that satisfy the requirements of all users
- simplifying systems and internal arrangements
- introducing realistic training programmes.

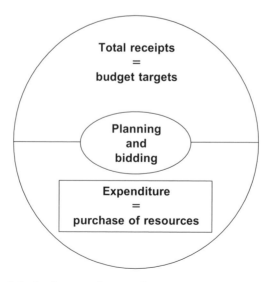

**Figure 1.2**  Receipts, budgets and expenditure.

# Project management

As the difficulties outlined above are complex, the application of a form of project management to one, some or all of the problem areas is a recommended format. Below is a checklist of project management terminology.

---

**Checklist of project management terminology and definitions**

▼   *Project.* This is usually a series of complex multidisciplinary management tasks that may span a protracted period, culminating in a single outcome (e.g. the closure or commissioning of a unit, the implementation of a new system, or in this case improvement in the quality of a financial or business process). One important characteristic of a project is its suitability for being divided into a number of stages that can be individually completed within a defined time frame.

▼   *Management.* There are many definitions, but in this case the one I favour is 'getting things done through people'.

▼   *Project board.* This consists of a small number of senior managers/ directors (often only two – in this case, representing finance and nursing) who are empowered to make decisions without referral upwards. The project board broadly specifies the problem(s), appoints the project manager, agrees the overall approach or project plan, receives reports, participates in end-stage assessments, and signs stages (or eventually, the whole project) off.

▼   *Project manager.* This individual is appointed by the project board from within the current cadre of suitable staff, and in the case of a major project he or she is formally seconded to the project for a specific period of time. The project manager prepares the project plan, obtains approval from the board, and keeps the board informed of progress.

▼   *Planning and mapping the process.* This mechanism seeks to represent graphically in the form of a map or outline critical path the intricacies of the sequence of events that have to fit together so that completion is achieved with minimum disruption within the agreed time scales. It is a useful technique that facilitates display where all members of the team can view and comment on the incidents.

▼   *Stages.* These must be easily identified as having a distinct beginning and a clearly recognisable end, so that when a stage is complete, there are no loose ends and a conclusion can be agreed.

▼ *Stage manager.* This function may be undertaken by the project manager, but usually if the project is large, a separate manager (who is responsible to the project manager) is appointed for each stage.

▼ *Quality assurance team.* Although they have to work within the corporate framework and towards the overall objectives, team members have a special interest in the validity, veracity, timeliness and sensitivity of tasks that are being investigated. For example, the quality assurance team would be deeply involved in identifying, testing and generally investigating data sources that will support various initiatives. It would also be involved in discussions and consultation with users.

▼ *Implementation team.* This team is responsible for the detailed main steps which are recognisable milestones along the implementation process. They should be tested by parallel running (see below) to determine whether they conform to this definition. In other words, when they are completed, will we clearly recognise this achievement?

▼ *Parallel running.* This is particularly valuable if new technology is being commissioned. It involves maintaining the old system in tandem with the new one, and comparing the results to ensure that all circumstances have been incorporated.

▼ *Walk through.* Again this technique is mainly used as new systems are being developed. It is a method of demonstrating how the new system will work by step-by-step explanation and example.

▼ *End-stage assessment.* This is carried out by the project board in conjunction with the project manager. When the stage has been satisfactorily completed, it is signed off and the next stage can be initiated.

▼ *Review.* This must be undertaken at regular intervals by the project manager to check that all aspects are up to speed, or if not, whether the whole project timetable can be amended to account for the variation.

▼ *Audit.* This function may be performed at any time, either in a peer group (as with medical audit) or in a more formal independent mode (where an outside assessor may be used to examine the project and make recommendations).

▼ *Signing off.* This is undertaken by the project board in conjunction with the project manager. It is the formal act of stage or project completion.

# Key stages

Key stages will vary from one project to another. For example, implementation may itself be a prolonged process and therefore might need to be treated as a project in its own right. With that reservation, Figure 1.3 illustrates how improvements in the quality of the processes outlined above might be tackled.

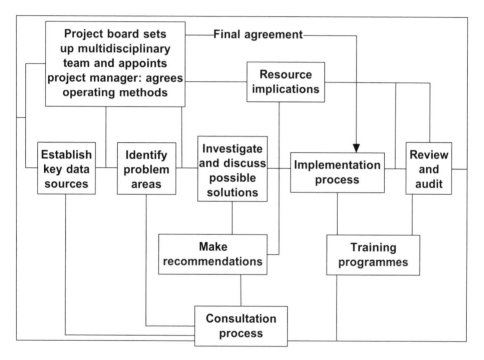

**Figure 1.3**  Key stages of project management.

Below is a checklist of the detailed work and data collection that are needed to support successful key stage management.

> **Checklist of key stage elements**
>
> ▼  *Key data sources and validity*. Although anecdotal evidence should not be relied upon, unsubstantiated impressions nevertheless highlight areas that merit investigation. Low morale is one pointer to poor quality processes. Establish a performance database for staff turnover, sickness, absenteeism, accidents, complaints, mistakes, fraud,

deliberate vandalism, etc. and any other untoward events, and obtain comparisons from similar departments and/or other organisations. Keep records of disciplinary matters. Assess the state of morale based on reliable data. An unacceptable level of losses, increases in the number of claims for negligence or non-compliance with contractual obligations are also indicators to which numbers can be attached and which can be verified.

▼ *Problem areas*. In terms of financial processes, problems can occur at any juncture and may even be caused by a different member of staff to the one who has to sort it out. However, apart from direct losses, whose existence is usually fairly obvious, other problems may continue unremarked so long as they are individually resolved in the short term. For example, if there is a problem at departmental level with regard to submitting overtime claims in time, so long as they are dealt with quickly when the pay deficiency comes to light, the individual member of staff is usually satisfied but the underlying cause may not be solved, resulting in continuing frustration and extra work in the payroll office.

▼ *Possible solutions*. The full range of options available to solve the problem(s) must be considered in a joint forum so that a mutual understanding is reached and a preferred option is identified.

▼ *Resource implications*. Although one of the key purposes of any process quality initiative is to cut down on waste, additional resources at the point of pressure must always be a consideration. Tangible and intangible benefits, together with the possible movement of resources, are therefore distinctly relevant to this stage (see hints below).

▼ *Consultation process*. In large-scale projects (e.g. where major change is contemplated), consultation will be a continuous arrangement involving clinical and allied disciplines, unions and staff associations, patients and relatives, public representatives, local contiguous authorities and organisations that are likely to be affected by the proposals. In recent times most public authorities have become quite adept at managing this process, but – cynically – there is always a suspicion that, to the public servant, consultation means simply providing information. Clearly a two-way dialogue is most beneficial, but this in turn causes problems. For example, where a particular point of view is contrary to the broad thrust of the organisation's strategy, what weight should be attributed to it (see hints below)?

▼ *Recommendations*. These must be based upon sound research, an appropriate consideration of all the options, and a robust methodology that favours one choice. Resource implications, training and any other relevant conditions should also be clearly stated.

▼  *Training programmes.* Where there is an established need (e.g. a new computerised system), programmes must be planned and implemented at appropriate times. They should not be merely an afterthought.

▼  *Final-stage assessment and agreement.* This is usually undertaken by the project board in consultation with the project manager. It is an act of completion that clearly signals the achievement of the primary goal. However, where implementation is a single stage, this may be inserted as final, i.e. the implementation stage becomes the final stage.

▼  *Implementation process.* Where more work has to be undertaken by way of implementation, the process itself may be broken down into stages and managed in accordance with the above descriptions.

▼  *Audit and review.* No change, however small, should be made by the project board without arranging for a regular independent audit and a frequent internal review by the board in conjunction with the project manager. In this way it is possible to assess the degree of satisfaction that is derived as a result of the project, and adjustments can be made as appropriate.

---

**Tips from the front office**

▼  Do not waste resources on a battle that you cannot win.
▼  If necessary, apologise, make reparation and regroup.
▼  Make sure that there is absolute uniformity and solidarity in approach.
▼  Bind members into cabinet-style commitment to the project.
▼  Sort out differences of feelings, facts and figures, together.

---

**Tip from the front office**

▼  Although most areas of this analysis can be easily costed, other benefits, etc. have to be taken into account. For situations where no weighting and scoring mechanism is in place, here is a method to get you started.
 – Make a comprehensive list of tasks to be measured.
 – Set out key criteria, safety, timeliness, veracity, etc.

- Score each criterion within a rating band of, say, one to five.
- Decide what each score indicates. For example, 1 = not good, 3 = acceptable, 5 = best practice.
- Add across to determine the overall rating.

# Case study

The initial results of the Balance of Care Scrutiny of care provided by St Bedeful Acute Hospital Trust found that there was up to 20% stagnation in the ability to manage the elderly care programme properly. The main points that were highlighted were as follows.

- There was a 17% stagnation rate in discharge potential, resulting in lost bed days.
- There also appeared to be an unnecessary 10% readmission rate due to inappropriate use of the existing discharge policy.
- There was a 19% or higher incidence of inappropriate admissions to care homes in the community.
- There was insufficient provision for respite care and rehabilitation.

These indicators are contrary to the legitimate emphasis on the need for increased independence through rehabilitation, and there was a compelling argument for a more integrated abundance of clinical, therapeutic, social and environmental rehabilitation interventions. Consequently, an integrated approach involving the local Social Services department has been developed for service arrangements to provide more suitable cost-effective alternatives to unnecessary hospital stays, care home arrangements and other expensive forms of care packages.

As a joint project, the old sanatorium building, now renamed 'Near-Home', has been refurbished and developed to facilitate the discharge of elderly patients/clients from one level of care and their admission to another lower and more appropriate level of care without the need to rush them into making life-changing decisions about their future. Operating through appropriate teams, it will be managed on a strict short-term-stay policy. It will also accommodate respite and rehabilitation services.

It is located in a pleasant setting, separated from the main St Bedeful's hospital complex by a small area of mature woodland. It was originally constructed as a sanatorium for patients suffering from tuberculosis. With the significant reduction in the incidence of that disease, the estate was transferred into the mainstream of healthcare in 1950, and was devoted to the care of the elderly until the effects of care in the community initiatives rendered it unnecessary.

Ms Nora Rightly, who has experience in the social care dimension and was previously a project manager, has been appointed as head of the new facility. The development of the joint project was managed in accordance with project management structure and method.

An outline of the structure and stages is shown in Figure 1.4.

Assessment and evaluation stages (which also involved the quality assurance group) have now been completed.

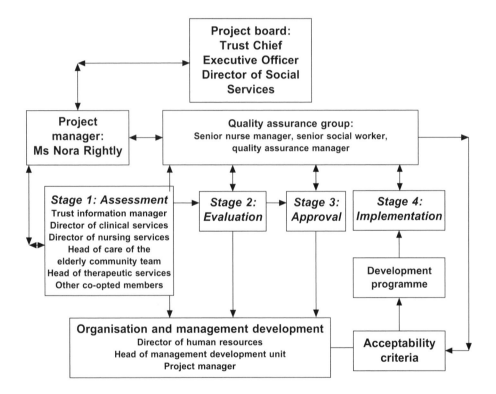

**Figure 1.4**   Near-Home facility joint project management: structure and stages.

# 2

# Gifts and hospitality

Frontline staff are frequently the first point of contact for a potential donor, but they may be unsure of the correct way to deal with that person who is waving a brown envelope. They may also be too busy to even contemplate either the beneficial effects of a genuine goodwill gesture, the ongoing running costs of a piece of equipment, or the more sinister implications of someone seeking to compromise the organisation. It seems so ungrateful either to hesitate or to refuse a gift that the prospect of public relations disaster can precipitate acceptance.

This chapter aims to:

- help managers to write a business protocol that will provide a consistent guide
- brief managers and frontline staff who have to advise prospective donors
- provide frontline staff with practical guidance where none is readily available
- assist in determining parameters for quality audit.

It clarifies specific issues such as the following:

- when a gift, sponsorship or hospitality can be accepted
- what other considerations have to be taken into account
- how a gift or hospitality should be accepted
- whether certain items may be retained for the individual's own use
- any other internal procedures.

After reading this chapter, you should have a good understanding of the following:

- context and issues relevant to the acceptance of gifts and hospitality
- value and goodwill inherent in gifts, legacies and endowments
- practical aspects of fundraising
- the need for communication and co-ordination
- principles and factors that influence the development of a code of good conduct
- an outline of procedures for frontline staff to follow.

# The issues

According to the popular cynical myth, there is no such thing as a free lunch. 'Beware of Greeks bearing gifts' is another well-known saying that embodies a note of caution against thoughtless acceptance. Even so, a gift is defined as that which is *voluntarily bestowed without expectation of return* (in legal terminology such a return is called a consideration).

There is no obligation to make any kind of reciprocal gesture. However, it is in the interests of beneficiaries for wise donors to *indicate their intentions in writing*. In the case of the transfer of all or part of an estate, a deed of transfer is required.

Gifts are usually given without condition. They are a recognition or token of esteem, kinship, friendship, etc., and are often symbolic. For example, the most famous gifts in Christendom — gold, frankincense and myrrh — are generally taken to signify kingship, religious or spiritual leadership, and an intimation of sorrow or an early death.

Before the inception of the NHS, hospital services relied heavily upon the generosity of better-off members of the general public. Many have endowed beds, wards and even hospitals through a straightforward transfer of funds or through legacies. In today's depressing financial climate this reservoir of goodwill is obviously a valuable source of alternative resource provision.

However, the acceptance of large-scale gifts, equipment, transport or property commits the organisation to running costs, maintenance and possible replacement. These factors, together with consultation with relevant professionals and analysis of the likely suitability and degree of utility of the proposed gift, need careful consideration.

It is also important to bear in mind the possibility that the acceptance of a gift may generate a conflict of interest with a health organisation's vision and purpose statements. At the very least the effect would be embarrassment, but clearly there may be more serious consequences. Perhaps the best-known example would be an association with the tobacco industry.

Below is a checklist of key issues.

---

**Checklist of key issues with regard to gifts**

▼   A gift of money or kind may appear to be the answer to funding problems, but donors can have other motives, especially where the gift is clearly intended for the recipient's personal use.

▼   Gifts can range from innocent promotional products to the sinister desire to exert undue external influence on the internal affairs of an organisation.

▼ Most readers will be aware of various scandals that have plagued public life.

▼ Although everyone is flattered by the offer of a gift or hospitality, care must be taken to ensure that acceptance does not compromise either the person or the organisation.

▼ On the other hand, lack of interest, prevarication or outright refusal of a gift by or on behalf of a health or social care organisation can cause considerable damage to its relationship with the community that it is supposed to interact with and serve.

▼ Many readers will have viewed with dismay the efforts of private citizens, filled with determination to raise funds for an item of medical equipment or otherwise provide a service that they have perhaps been told would have saved the life of a loved one, come to an inexplicable standstill.

▼ This may have been due to internal constraints (e.g. the cost of running the equipment), its continued appropriateness, or perhaps the fact that events have overtaken its utility.

▼ Therefore it is important to maintain communication with the donor and the public at large so that insensitive bureaucracy is not blamed.

# The establishment of acceptability criteria

As with clinical and other areas, a framework for the establishment of acceptability criteria will be of great assistance in situations where there is the potential for conflict between a donor's proposals, the organisation's culture or perceived need and running costs. An outline structure within which everyone may work and resolve difficulties without creating further problems is illustrated in Figure 2.1.

In this outline the essential relationships that govern the way in which the gifting process is managed are characterised by agreement and bridging of the communication gap.

## Agreement

When reaching a consensus between management, frontline staff and prospective donors, the following key points have to be considered.

- *Utility.* Here the donor's intentions with regard to the type and purpose of the gift must be discreetly tested to ensure that it will not only fulfil a

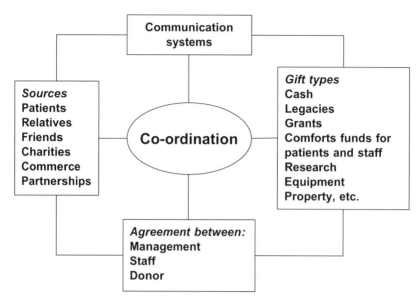

**Figure 2.1**   Outline of structure for gifts management.

need but will be consistently useful for the foreseeable future. In other words, efforts should be made to ensure that donors (e.g. patients' relatives) are not responding to a very limited perception of need. If this is the case, donors must be steered away from being specific and towards a more general expression of intention that is more flexible.

- *Appropriateness*. The proposed gift must be consistent with the profile of the unit where it will be used. This means that there must be internal consultation with concerned professionals.
- *Costs*. Making the best use of any addition to a department may result in a significant increase in resource commitment. For example, the acceptance of an electric organ in a care home for the elderly implies that to conform with utility criteria, there would be a member of staff with keyboard skills who would be available at reasonable intervals.
- *Harmony*. Acceptance should always be made dependent on perceived legal, moral and ethical considerations and limitations.

# Bridging the communication gap

A donor may specify that a gift of property or money is to be used directly for a particular project (e.g. the immediate purchase of a piece of equipment). In other cases where there is no such expressed intention, property may be retained as an investment and the income used for the purpose specified.

Usually gifts of money are kept in trust and invested so that a source of semi-permanent income is maintained. However, the following factors are relevant.

- In larger health and social care organisations, a gap can develop between the donor, local staff and the actual commissioning and use of the gift, particularly where funding has to be converted into the practical item.
- Further complications can occur where older specific funds, because of modernisation, closures, etc., can no longer be used for their original purpose.

In order to avoid the development of a communication gap between donor, organisation and frontline staff, it is necessary to have in place a system of regular information sharing so that all interested parties are kept up to date. This involves the co-ordination of a variety of initiatives, which include the development of protocols governing the acceptance of gifts and hospitality, and practical guidance for frontline staff and managers.

# Case study

Friends and Parents of Young Disabled Adults (FAPYDA), in consultation with Nora Rightly, the head of the rehabilitation complex, decided to raise funds to buy an adult-size rocking-horse. The proceeds from various events were entrusted to Ms Rightly, who with the agreement of the St Bedeful's treasurer, Midas Luckpenny, regularly lodged the money at the cashier's office to a specific Rocking-Horse Account.

When FAPYDA had accumulated sufficient money, because it was believed that the trust had better access to the marketplace through its supplies department and was therefore in a good position to 'do a deal', FAPYDA decided to ask the trust to process an order for the rocking-horse and to pay for it from the identified fund. Nora Rightly hoped that when the rocking-horse was delivered, the FAPYDA chairman, Mr Smith, would make a presentation of the gift at a suitably organised occasion to which the press would be invited. By this means it was hoped that all those involved would benefit from a certain amount of favourable publicity.

Unfortunately, Midas Luckpenny was on holiday when the request to purchase the rocking-horse arrived at St Bedeful's front office, where no one else seemed to be conversant with the details. This was only the start of a long list of embarrassing problems.

- Authority to purchase was delayed until Ms Rightly enquired about progress.

- Then, after much explanation, the accounts staff announced that the rocking-horse account had insufficient funds.
- The FAPYDA chairman had a record of the amounts handed over to Ms Rightly, but she was unable to produce all of her receipts.
- After some acrimony and finger pointing, but just before the police were called, the accounts staff discovered that the money had been erroneously credited to three separate accounts – Rocking-Horse account, the Horse account and FAPYDA.
- With some reservations, approval to purchase was finally given, but the supplies manager, evangelised by a series of enlightening value-for-money seminars, subjected the rocking-horse request to scrutiny with regard to the efficacy of such a purchase, and pointed out to Mr Smith that a number of smaller rocking-horses could have been purchased for less money.
- Again the Chief Executive Officer (CEO) had to intervene.
- In order to save face, the supplies manager, who everyone had to agree was only doing his job, then proceeded to impose an inappropriately prolonged contracting process.
- This resulted in further strong words from Mr Smith, who had 'lost faith entirely', but he calmed down when he received an unexpected invitation to become one of St Bedeful's honorary governors.
- Everyone agreed that the arrival of the rocking-horse had been well worth the long wait, and all were equally impressed with the hospitality bestowed at the Grand Gifting Ceremony – a real cucumber sandwich and green-leaf tea affair.
- What a pity that even the fond memory of that glittering event was spoiled when a few days later Mr Smith received a substantial bill for the food –*not that much surely*.
- Apparently the catering contractor had not been properly briefed about the precise nature of the internal funding arrangements that the CEO had in mind. More excuses and apologies followed.

## What went wrong?

According to the Internal Inquiry Team, chaired by Midas Luckpenny, blame could not be attributed to any single person. Instead, the team was inclined toward the view that the system was deficient. Accordingly, the ancient upright manual Imperial typewriter on which the offending 'bill' had been typed was condemned in favour of a new integrated computerised catering information system. The typewriter was later ceremoniously destroyed in a typewriter-throwing contest that was held during a fundraising family fun day at the Near-Home facility.

However, some time afterwards it came to light that the old Imperial had been a gift from a famous author and, because of its interesting provenance, had a considerable antique value. This matter is now being eagerly pursued by the press and the local MP.

# Guiding protocol principles

All organisations should develop guidelines that indicate acceptable limits within which staff may accept a gift.

# Specific considerations

## External influences

- *Legality*: make sure that offering or accepting the gift does not infringe the law.
- *Ethics*: check that there is no conflict of interest or damage to integrity (everyone is aware of the smoking habit/tobacco industry connection, but there are many other more subtle factors).
- *Equity*: test whether the gift is targeted at an individual or group within an organisation.
- *Intention*: ensure that the offer or acceptance of the gift cannot be interpreted as a bribe.

## Internal constraints

- *Appropriateness*: a proposed gift must be appropriate to the strategic requirements of the recipient organisation.
- *Revenue consequences*: expensive equipment (e.g. scanners) inevitably incurs ongoing costs, and these must be carefully considered before accepting a gift.
- *Utility and obsolescence*: the proposed gift must have a realistic utility for the organisation.
- *Non-specific gifts or gifts of money*: if these are not limited to one specific purpose and have more general application, they provide managers with greater flexibility but this should not compromise the donor's reasonable intention.

# Co-ordination

A designated senior manager or director should have responsibility for co-ordinating various interests (e.g. clinical considerations, public relations, supply chain management, finance, total quality management).

# Acceptable promotional material

- Genuine marketing material (e.g. calendars, diaries, pencils) aimed at penetrating the workplace and maintaining existing market connections by creating genuine goodwill.
- Corporate hospitality to launch or renew interest in a product.
- Special customers' staff discount schemes.
- Sponsorship for sporting events and charitable fundraising.

# Communication and review

This must be undertaken in both promoting and accepting organisations.

# Practical steps for frontline staff and heads of departments

The offer of a gift often occurs at the most inopportune moments. For example:

- when a staff member is unsure of the correct procedure
- in clinical areas where patients' needs have to take priority
- when senior managers are not available to give advice
- in busy departments where there is too little time available to pay full attention to that person in the corridor who is waving a brown envelope.

The checklist below provides guidance, *but should never override the authority's own regulations.*

---

**Checklist of possible acceptability criteria**

▼ Ensure that prospective donors are treated politely.
▼ Ask them to wait in a suitable area until they can receive proper attention.
▼ If possible, make sure that the most senior member of staff interviews them.

▼ Interviews should take place in a private space and without inter-ruption.

▼ Take notes of the donor's intentions.

▼ If in doubt, do not accept the offer of any personal gift or hospital-ity without reference to a senior manager.

▼ Avoid indicating acceptance of very specific gifts for use within your organisation, but try to be encouraging. Refer any such cases to senior management as soon as possible.

▼ Issue a receipt for any cash or cheques received.

▼ Keep cash in secure receptacles — *not* in desk drawers or filing cabi-nets (*see* Chapter 3).

▼ Observe strict rules about keys to safe places (*see* Chapter 3).

▼ Make sure that all monies are lodged with the cashier at the earliest opportunity (*see* Chapter 3).

▼ Donors should always be officially thanked by letter (signed by the designated officer).

▼ Maintain an up-to-date register of all gifts offered and received.

▼ Make sure that you receive regular reports on accumulated funds.

▼ Maintain the right to influence spending.

---

**Tips from the front office**

Remember the seven P's when dealing with prospective donors.

▼ *Politeness*: make sure that the prospective donor is respected.

▼ *Privacy*: provide seclusion for proper discussion.

▼ *Purpose*: ensure that you grasp the donor's full intentions.

▼ *Prevarication*: always play for time to obtain advice.

▼ *Proof of transaction*: ensure that receipts are written.

▼ *Protection*: a gift of cash needs to be kept secure until it can be banked.

▼ *Performance record*: always send a letter of thanks.

In cases where large and possibly over-generous gifts are offered for staff use, it is sometimes considered preferable to accept them subject to the gift being shared among staff or perhaps raffled for some charit-able purpose.

# 3

# Cash and security matters

In industry and commerce, companies regularly report losses of up to 3–5% of their turnover. Incidents range from inventory theft and forgery to bribes. Around 75% of these actions are committed by employees, a large proportion of which is due to collusion (two or more employees in key positions co-operating). Recognition of this serious problem, which also affects health and social care organisations, must be matched by increased awareness and the capability to eradicate the causes.

In the case of cash, despite the growing reliance upon credit cards and other methods used to transact business, there is still an amazing amount of cash or its equivalent in circulation in hospital and other health or social care environments.

The purposes for which cash is used vary widely. They range from cash-points to canteen and shop receipts, telephone and vending-machine takings, patients' and clients' monies and sales of produce (e.g. occupational therapy items). It must be remembered that where automated vending based on tokens has been introduced, usually cash must be used to obtain the tokens. Prevention of losses, and detection, investigation and maximisation of the recovery process must be priorities.

After reading this chapter you will be fully aware of the competences required to:

- receive, record and keep cash safely until it can be officially lodged
- be alert to the temptation that arises from too casual an approach to stock and equipment management
- take appropriate action in the case of suspected fraud or following a robbery
- manage fundraising so that high standards of accountability are achieved
- handle and manage patients' and clients' monies in a professional manner.

# The issues

Due to its convenient transportability and often also its ready availability, there are many difficulties and dangers inherent in the use of money. These include mistakes, negligence, robbery and fraud. Even though a particular aspect may be an outside contractor's responsibility, it must be borne in mind that the total volumes at a bank outlet or cashier's office may attract unwanted attention. These types of general risks to all personnel and visitors must be minimised.

Risks of loss and wastage occur as a direct result of not following the procedure that has been laid down (e.g. failure to control the movement of stock and items of equipment properly, or the need in certain situations, such as emptying a telephone box, to have a second person corroborate the amount of cash taken or the amount of stock delivered). Lack of attention to the processes of checking, recording, safe keeping and/or banking the money can also cause problems. Figure 3.1 illustrates the correct sequence of events for receiving cash.

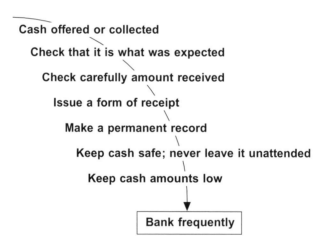

**Figure 3.1**   Outline procedure for receiving cash.

The key issues that arise from this are listed below.

---

**Checklist of points to remember when handling cash**

▼   When money is *offered or collected*, it sometimes happens that it is not the correct or expected amount. It is good practice to check this out at the time rather than later on or, worse still, not at all! The main although not exclusive occasions when this occurs are:

      – settlement of a debt – check the debtors register

      – clearance of a cash till – check and make a record of the till or audit roll

      – clearing cash from a vending machine or telephone box – check and record the reading on the audit counter.

▼ Always *count* the cash carefully *in the presence of a second person* who can corroborate the amount received. If you are not sure of the amount, take your time and don't panic. Count it all again. Always get the second person to *check and counter-sign the record.*

▼ If you are receiving a cheque, check the following:

      – date (especially the year if it is the beginning of a new year)

      – the amount in words should agree with the figures

      – the signature – and check that two signatures are not required

      – the cheque should be crossed A/C payee.

▼ Write a *receipt* indicating the correct amount received and the purpose for which it was received.

▼ Make a *permanent record*. Usually receipts are written in duplicate, so the copy in the receipt book will be satisfactory.

▼ Keep cash *safe* at all times and never leave it unattended.

▼ Keep records separate from cash.

▼ To avoid temptation, *maintain low levels of cash* (e.g. only petty cash).

▼ Bank cash frequently and always obtain a receipt from the bank!

---

**Checklist of basic principles and tips**

Cash will do nicely, thank you …

*Don't*

▼ Take cash from strangers – make sure that you know the identity of the person who is making the offer and the precise nature of their business (*see* Chapter 2). Be polite, but:

      – find out the business of a potential benefactor

      – anticipate a hidden and unethical agenda.

▼ Accept a gift for an unrealistic purpose.

▼ Accept a personal gift or act on behalf of a colleague.

▼ Leave cash unattended.

*Do*

▼ Always keep cash in secure receptacles, preferably a safe.

▼ Avoid using desk drawers, filing cabinets, etc.

▼ Observe strict rules about keys to safe places.

▼ Count cash in the presence of the benefactor or a witness to corroborate the amount.

▼   Keep a record and keep it separate from the cash box.
▼   Write a receipt.
▼   Keep cash levels low.
▼   Make regular lodgements.
▼   In the case of a gift, ensure that an official letter of thanks is dispatched.
▼   Make sure that you receive regular reports on accumulated funds.
▼   Maintain the right to influence spending.

---

**Tips from the front office**

▼   Treat cash with respect.
▼   Think of cash as being too hot to handle.
▼   Regard cash as a dangerous substance.
▼   Keep it locked up.

## What to do if you suspect stealing or pilfering

- Do not act immediately on an instinct, or in response to gossip or a feeling about cash or items that appear to be missing.
- Collect hard evidence (e.g. consistent discrepancies in stock levels, deliveries, cash shortages, etc.).
- Seek an explanation from the staff member responsible.
- When you are satisfied, report the matter to your senior officer.
- Make sure that you retain a record of all that was reported.
- Co-operate fully with the subsequent investigation.
- Expect to shoulder some of the blame for not being rigorous enough.
- Arrange for all of the relevant locks to be changed.

## What to do if you are faced with a robber who is demanding money or other items by threatening you

- Do not panic.
- In no circumstances should you put yourself at risk.
- Comply with the robber's instructions.

- Do not try to tackle the robber(s).
- Do not run after the robber(s) while they make their escape.
- Raise the alarm.
- Note the names of any witnesses.
- Write down as detailed a description as you can remember, including the number of individuals, their heights, colour, accent, etc.
- Check losses.

# Managing patient/client monies

There are times when the management of cash extends beyond the receipt of money. These include certain payments, such as patients' or clients' private property. Although it is desirable for patients and clients to maintain their independence, it may be that because of infirmity or a lack of secure premises, patients and clients need their cash to be handled on their behalf.

In order to avoid allegations of mismanagement, it is essential that private property transactions are conducted in a businesslike and professional manner. Below is a short list of safeguards that will protect the interests of both the patient or client and the frontline member of staff or manager.

---

**Checklist of main considerations with regard to patient/client money management**

▼ Form a Committee of Oversight consisting of senior professionals who are concerned with patients' or clients' welfare.

▼ Ensure that all monies are lodged to a bank account.

▼ Seek advice on investment thresholds.

▼ Keep a reasonable cash float, topped up from a bank account, to deal with emergencies.

▼ Maintain a cash requisitioning duplicate book system for withdrawals from patient or client accounts, with proper methods of signature and counter-signature together with spending details.

▼ Keep all receipts with cash requisition for later inspection.

▼ Check cash and bank funds regularly, and present accounts to an oversight committee on a regular basis (e.g. every quarter).

▼ Appoint an independent auditor to conduct an annual detailed audit.

---

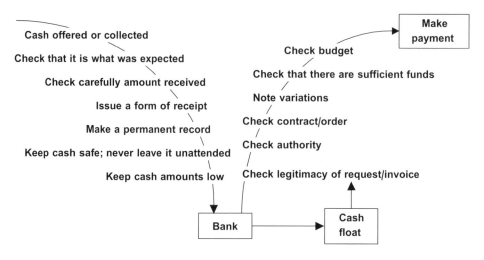

**Figure 3.2** Receiving cash and making a payment.

The process of making a payment from cash is illustrated in Figure 3.2. It can be used, for example, in the case of patients' or clients' personal monies or fundraising, as the principles are more or less the same.

The main areas that require attention are listed below.

- *Request/requisition/invoice*. No payment process should ever be initiated without the receipt of a demand in a recognisable form.
- *Authority*. Check that the original 'deal' was negotiated at the correct level of authority.
- *Contractor or order*. If this is appropriate, check that all of the details coincide.
- *Variations in quality, quantity or previously agreed price*. These are matters for concern.
- *Sufficient funds*. In all cases, embarrassment can be avoided by checking that adequate funds are available to cover a cash withdrawal.
- *Budget*. Where appropriate, make sure that budget provision has not been exceeded.
- *Payment*. This should only be made when you are completely satisfied.

# Fundraising

Those who become involved in fundraising for charitable purposes need to be aware of the problems that can and frequently do arise from large-scale cash handling. They must take steps to reduce the risks both to themselves and to the organisation that they represent.

Although genuine mistakes can and do occur, it is essential that, as far as possible, fundraisers are protected from accusations of negligence or misappropriation, and that members and beneficiaries are assured of efficient and appropriate cash management.

Fundraisers must recognise their accountability to the umbrella organisation, the general public and prospective beneficiaries. They must also take reasonable precautions to demonstrate their good stewardship. This means starting the way they intend to go on.

Fundraisers must get things right from the organisation's inception. This means preparing the ground for an accurate record of money that flows into the organisation, and ensuring that authorised payments have proper supporting documentation for later inspection.

Fundraisers must:

- agree upon an adequate structure to provide credibility
- abide by a few simple rules to ensure integrity
- adopt acceptable methods of record keeping to render an accurate account.

Below are several checklists that will help those who are contemplating fundraising to put in place arrangements that will stand up to later scrutiny. These are as follows:

- formation of a steering group
- organisation of a public meeting
- development of a constitution.

---

**Checklist of tasks relating to the formation of a steering group**

▼  Define the purpose of the group and decide upon a name (e.g. Friends of Special Care Baby Unit (SCBU)).

▼  Make sure that neither the purpose nor the name appears to conflict with the title or the objectives of another like-minded group.

▼  Obtain the support of relevant professional(s).

▼  Inform your manager, the Chief Executive and the Treasurer of your intentions.

▼  If possible, take any advice that is offered (e.g. take note of the acceptability criteria; *see* Chapter 2).

▼  Buy a receipt book and raffle tickets.
▼  Make a list of interested people who would be enthusiastic enough to become members of a steering group.
▼  Select about ten individuals on the basis of:
   − *functionality* − experience of finance, administration, public relations or marketing
   − *inclusivity* − patients, relatives and members of the general public form this group of candidates, but be sure to take into account the general make-up of the population so as not to discriminate in favour of any particular colour or creed.
▼  The purpose of the steering group is to:
   − decide the overall strategy and agenda for a later public meeting
   − agree a small membership fee (say £5) as a seed fund
   − gather together feasible fundraising ideas
   − draft a constitution (see below).
▼  Do not waste time − collect the membership fee from the steering group before the members leave.
▼  Write a receipt for each subscription as you collect it.
▼  Obtain official approval for the use of a photocopier − the usual fee may be waived for a good cause.

---

**Checklist for first public meeting**

▼  Obtain the support of local papers and obtain free publicity for the first public meeting.
▼  Post a notice about the public meeting in suitable shops and offices and on noticeboards.
▼  At the public meeting:
   − make a presentation in which you give brief details and indicate funding targets for the first year, second year, etc.
   − introduce each member of the steering group and give them a minute or two to indicate their background and interest in the project (you hope that later they will be elected as office bearers or committee members)
   − persuade one or more professionals to speak about the need for the proposed project
   − outline the way forward.
▼  Approve the constitution (see below).
▼  Seek ideas from the floor on fundraising events.
▼  Elect a chairperson, secretary, treasurer and committee.

▼   Obtain agreement on a membership fee.

▼   Help the newly elected treasurer to collect the membership fee.

▼   Write receipts for each subscription.

▼   Hold a raffle to augment seed funds.

▼   Agree a date, time and venue for the next meeting to agree detailed proposals for fundraising.

▼   After the public meeting, open a bank account with a local bank that offers free banking services. Take advice from the trust treasurer, and lodge all monies collected. Do not forget:

  − a new account will require two signatures

  − sample signatures of all approved signatories will be required

  − proof of identification will be needed − check with the bank first.

---

**Checklist of main financial considerations relating to a constitution**

▼   *Name*: for example − St Bedeful's Scanner Appeal Association.

▼   The association shall be non-political and non-sectarian. It shall not discriminate in favour of any person on the grounds of sex, colour or creed.

▼   *Purpose*: to raise funds by public subscription, fundraising events, sponsorship and any other appropriate arrangement over a period of two years.

▼   *Fund target*: £2 million.

▼   *Membership*: shall be open to all those interested in helping to raise money for this cause. Remember the association's commitment to equality above all else, and make sure that the choice of management team and committee demonstrates that commitment.

▼   *Management team*: a basic management team shall consist of a chairperson, secretary and treasurer. A vice-chairperson, assistant secretary and assistant treasurer can be added as appropriate to cover sickness, holidays, etc. However, it is more effective to keep numbers low.

▼   *Committee*: usually six committee members are sufficient, but in order to comply with inclusivity and equality it might be sensible to increase or decrease this number accordingly. Make provision for the inclusion of co-opted members who may have specialist skills or knowledge.

▼   *How a decision is reached*:

  − it is important that the management team and the committee have a unity of purpose

  − it follows therefore that when taking a decision, everyone − even if they are not in total agreement − will acquiesce

> - a simple majority with a strongly dissenting minority may lead to a split in the organisation
> - the chairperson, who may have a second or casting vote, nevertheless needs to have the patience to attain a position of consensus
> - where complete agreement is not possible, it may be necessary to refer the matter back to all of the members rather than risk an organisational split.
>
> ▼ *Term*: a three-year term for the management team and committee is usual.
>
> ▼ *Annual general meeting*: the rules governing the date upon which this event is to take place (usually on or near the anniversary of the first public meeting) need to be set down.
>
> ▼ *Bank account*: the management of the bank account (two signatories, etc.) needs to be spelt out.
>
> ▼ *Budget management and rules governing spending*: these should be made to comply with the outline rules mentioned above. The individuals who have authority to incur expenditure (make sure it is not the treasurer) also need to be stipulated and major items recorded as having been approved in the committee minutes.
>
> ▼ *Presentation and publication of accounts*: this usually takes place on an annual basis to coincide with the annual general meeting.
>
> ▼ *Auditor*: an independent auditor should be appointed.
>
> ▼ *Winding up of the association*: in the event of the association's purpose either being fulfilled or having no hope of fulfilment, the details of what should happen to any funds that have been collected need to be agreed.

# General improvements to an organisation's security

## Strategy

This defines the corporate attitude to fraud and facilitates control of the security dimension.

## Organisation

- Maintain independence of specialist functions to prevent collusion (two or more staff and/or a supplier needed to receive money, enter a contract or make a payment).

- Encourage the development of specialist financial and business teams.
- Structure teams to ensure that there is a consistent internal checking mechanism.
- Establish a separate security monitoring function and vigorously follow up discrepancies.

## Systems

- Utilise the latest data-mining and computer technology.
- Be aware of vulnerable areas, such as cash transfer points and stores.
- Protect audit trails and introduce efficient tracking systems.
- Remember that deleted data may still be recovered from the computer hard disk.
- Forensic accounting techniques should be appropriately deployed.

## Internal procedures

- Reduce all areas that might give rise to temptation.
- Ensure that a satisfactory internal check programme is maintained.
- Co-operate fully with internal and external audit.
- It is easier to make up an under-payment than to recover an over-payment.

## Response plan

This should include the following:

- what action to take (including disciplinary action)
- who to inform internally (e.g. directors, security, etc.) and externally (e.g. the police)
- how to maximise recovery
- particular weaknesses should be identified
- remedial action and review processes
- implementation of improvements.

---

**Tips from the front office**

▼ Be aware of the motivation (which is sometimes perverse) for fraud.
▼ Become familiar with the backgrounds of key staff members.

▼ Take steps to protect information sources.
▼ Forensic software can be used without the knowledge of an employee.
▼ Thoroughly investigate all complaints, and audit criticism.

# Case study

During the fundraising Family Fun Day that was held in the grounds of St Bedeful's Near-Home facility, thieves gained entry to Ms Nora Rightly's office through an open window. They found the keys to the safe (which they emptied) in an unlocked drawer. The detective constable was convinced that the thieves were opportunists, but her senior told her to use a bit of common sense.

'No fingerprints, you see. And didn't they take all the records? So we can't be sure exactly how much was missing. No, it was planned and it was an insider. Look at the evidence.' And the police managed to make all those who had access to either the office or the keys feel uncomfortable.

It was unfortunate that before any locks could be changed the thieves returned, presumably through the normal means of entry, and cleared Ms Rightly's office of its furniture, filing cabinet and personal computer.

# 4

# Planning essentials

Managers and frontline staff need to comprehend their fundamental influence over their internal consumption of resources in order to provide services to the external environment. Whether they are in commissioning or providing mode, in order to improve their own environmental conditions everyone must work to a plan for their department or unit – or their own individual development, for that matter. However, this is often counter-productive if their intentions are contrary to the thrust of the organisation's overall objectives.

Successful managers and frontline staff must have a good understanding of where they stand in the overall context, and are therefore well placed to take advantage of perceived opportunities. A grasp of both planning terminology and the general direction of the organisation will be of assistance to all those who are seeking to improve their prospects.

This chapter will help managers and frontline staff to comprehend the complexities of planning so that they can function in the correct planning mode when they wish to make significant improvements in their ward, department or unit.

After reading this chapter you will be able to plan more effectively for yourself and your department, through reference to the following checklists:

- factors that influence change
- fundamental features of a plan
- main external environmental influences
- ward/departmental/unit strengths, weaknesses, opportunities and threats.

## The issues

'Planning and development' is a familiar phrase which has firmly established the connection in the minds of most people between preparation for and maturity of an activity or group of activities. In planning terms, development must be interpreted in the context of change. Some form of planning is an essential feature of successful endeavour, even though there may not be much evidence of its existence. For example, at a basic level, plans may be little more than barely discernible patterns of behaviour which have been established through previous experience. However, where organisation is concerned planning has to be more complex and dedicated.

Many plans are inert in character – for example, those which are made in order to cover the most unlikely situations imaginable. Some plans are dormant and are activated only in specific, clearly defined circumstances (e.g. wills whose effect depends upon the demise of the testator). Other types of plans are designed for active use and are therefore not so dependent on confidentiality. Indeed it can be argued that in a more complex organisation, adherence to a plan can best be achieved through openness.

Planning processes reconcile the purpose or objective with the most efficient use of resources. In planning terms, two sets of basic data are therefore required. One set is concerned with the requirements of the external environment, and in this context managers need to be able to influence their external environment for the better. The other more familiar set is dedicated to the internal efficiency of the workplace. Here the performance of *all* resources must be considered. Through this process, a policy emerges that will be the main determining factor for immediate and future activity.

As far as health and social care organisations are concerned, although planning mechanisms at every stage are generally robust and scrupulous, the detail and sequence of events often appear remote to frontline managers and staff. However, ignorance of this key management function only causes them frustration when their endeavours to develop and create improvements appear contrary to the general direction of their host organisation.

Fortunately for those managers who wish to improve their position, although we live in a climate of continuous and unrelenting change, the factors that generate change (*see* checklist below) are consistent.

---

**Checklist of factors that influence change**

▼ Developments in clinical practice, new technology and scientific discovery leading to a much broader spectrum of available treatments and care arrangements.
▼ An ageing population that requires increasing support and care.
▼ Increasing patient/relative/client expectations and demand, and increasing patient/client numbers.
▼ Pressures arising from legal, ethical and moral judgements resulting from the application or otherwise of advances in the ability to care for and treat patients with conditions that had previously proved difficult or impossible to treat.

▼   Unacceptable waiting times and length of waiting lists, including the length of time patients/clients have to spend in waiting areas.
▼   A climate of near-zero financial growth.
▼   The need to further reduce costs, make savings and increase income.
▼   Continued alteration in the balance of care in favour of care in the community (e.g. bed blockers in the acute sector, and children possibly awaiting adoption in care homes in the childcare sector).

# Fundamental features of a plan

**Checklist of fundamental features of a plan**

▼   It embraces the suspension or reduction of one thing in favour of another.
▼   The movement in direction can result in turbulence both in reaction to announced changes and in retrospect.
▼   Nevertheless, a constant factor is the expected improvement in condition.
▼   It can therefore be argued that development covers all those arrangements which are embraced within the plan.
▼   The purpose of the traditional model is to create a reasonably permanent framework within which services can be delivered.
▼   Planning assumptions with regard to demography, geography, morbidity and mortality are usually broadly based, and forecasts of resource allocations may also seem vague. This is why much of the language in these documents is not very definitive.
▼   Nevertheless, planning implies progress towards achievable goals.
▼   It promotes a sense of security in continuity and improvement.
▼   The intention is to foster belief that the end product will in some way be better.
▼   Care must be taken to ensure that expectations are reasonable, to avoid dissatisfaction.
▼   There must therefore be a degree of flexibility to accommodate occasions when performance differs from the plan.
▼   Contingency quotients facilitate some revision.
▼   The plan must therefore be evolutionary in nature.

The elements to be considered are the main external and internal environmental influences that tend to limit the extent of a particular management role

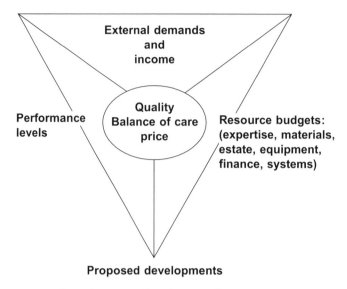

**Figure 4.1**   Reconciling the internal and external environments.

in both commissioning and providing care and treatment. Figure 4.1 illustrates the overall position.

# Gaining a sense of direction

There is little chance of a proposed development succeeding where there is a critical mass of external factors ranged against it. For example, if Government policy favours community-based initiatives for certain treatments or care, then there is little chance of a development that is not amenable to that kind of approach. Similarly, if departmental or commissioner preference directs funding towards other schemes, managers whose services are not so favoured must consider their options.

However, this does not mean that because external opinion is against a particular proposal, managers must abandon a cherished scheme. Instead, they must seek to create an external climate in which their proposals will have a better chance. They must learn to manage their external environment.

Below is a checklist of the main external influences.

---

**Checklist of main external environmental influences**

▼   Commissioner requirements for services to patients and clients.
▼   Sources and regulators of finance.

▼ The market in terms of patients and clients.
▼ Suppliers in terms of physical resources.
▼ Sources of income, including statutory funding.
▼ Relevant ministerial and Government departmental contacts.
▼ Statutory regulators and commentators, including the Audit Commission and arm's-length inspection units.
▼ Patient and client support groups, including individual benefactors.
▼ Collegiate support, including staff and professional associations.
▼ Coterminous commissioners and providers, including the voluntary sector.
▼ Other influential factors, including local authority membership, MPs, the media, etc.

# Being informed

The information that forms the basis for planning is progressively enriched and enhanced through operation and activity originating from strategic direction. It is therefore possible to develop the structure outlined in Figure 4.2 to account for greater complexity.

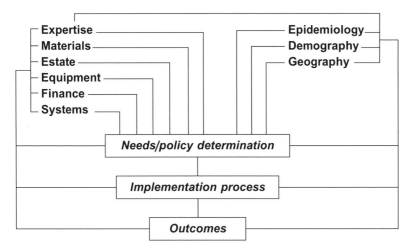

**Figure 4.2**   Planning information.

# Analysis

In this context, SWOT or TOWS analysis should assist the planning process. When TOWS analysis is applied, strengths and weaknesses are regarded

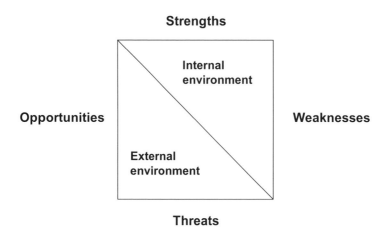

**Figure 4.3** Historical evaluation.

mainly as internal environmental characteristics, and opportunities and threats exist externally. Thus a matrix can be developed that analyses these factors over time (*see* Figure 4.3).

Below is a set of sample checklists that will assist managers in beginning to list in a systematic way those areas and elements which may need attention. These sample checklists cannot be exclusive. They are *for guidance only*, and are intended to stimulate managers to tailor their plans to fit their individual circumstances.

---

**Checklist of strengths**

▼ *Traditional values*:
  – reputation as a provider to the external environment
  – competence in a range of specialist services
  – manageably safe volumes of care and treatments.
▼ *Quality*:
  – development of identifiable standards and protocols
  – valid measurement techniques in operation
  – improvements identified and attainable within time scales.
▼ *Current workloads and dependencies*:
  – current trends within safe limits and capable of expansion
  – service developments compatible with available resources.
▼ *Resources (GEESE)*: here we are looking for flexibility and the potential to make a better match between patient and client use and the consumption of resources. We want to see enough spare capacity to cope with changes that will be necessary as the plan is developed.

1 *Goods and services*:
   – developments in procurement arrangements
   – utility in the use of purchasing power
   – improvements in materials, logistics and management
   – reduction in stocks held.

2 *Expertise*:
   – organisation that is easily understood and amenable to change
   – manageable turnover rates
   – healthy spread across age groups, gender and cultural origin
   – staff support facilities that encourage development.

3 *Estate*:
   – good-quality grounds, buildings and services
   – manageable maintenance packages
   – identification of vacant or low-usage building stock
   – estate rationalisation proposals.

4 *Systems*:
   – movements towards the implementation and satisfactory development of all major systems.

5 *Equipment*:
   – identification of good-condition, up-to-date equipment
   – listing of equipment that is under-utilised, with a view to rationalisation.

▼ *Development*: developments are the most attractive form of planning, but in a financial growth climate of near zero, advances can usually only be contemplated when a movement or recognisable surplus in resource capacity has been identified. Usually this is only possible where resource mobility has been created – in other words, there is reduction or retraction of one service in favour of another.

▼ *Financial position*:
   – sound financial infrastructure with demonstrably capable budget managers
   – scope for redistribution and mobility within a realistic financial plan.

---

### Checklist of possible weaknesses

▼ *Visible quality deficits*: deficiencies in quality of life are apparent in the population profiles of the population served. Health and social service managers recognise and compare these with the problems that they have to deal with. For example, on a national level:

   – life expectancy at birth is 74 years for men and 79 years for women
   – the birth rate is about 13 per 1000
   – there are 5000 infant deaths in a population of 59 million
   – deaths under 1 year of age occur in 6 in 1000 live births
   – the total death rate per 1000 is 10.7.

▼  *Regulatory or audit findings (health, safety and other regulations)*: a key
   requirement is to adhere to all regulations and advice to ensure
   the health and safety of patients, clients, staff and members of the
   general public. Where any part of an operation has been found to be
   in any respect defective, managers will be taking steps to rectify
   the situation. However, where a major problem has been identified
   (e.g. evidence of extensive use of asbestos cladding), then the impact
   on service commissioning and provision in that area will be affected,
   and that effect will have to be included in the business plan.

▼  *External audit*: the main sources of significant influence stem from
   the Comptroller and Auditor General, whose reports to Parliament
   may be the cause of select committee questions to the relevant
   officials. The results of these investigations are often the forerunner
   of amendments and adjustments to the way in which business is
   conducted. Value-for-money (VFM) scrutinies that cover a range of
   activities are examples of the type of topic under consideration. The
   results of some of these are quite well known (e.g. recruitment and
   advertising, residential accommodation, non-emergency ambulance
   service, central stores policy, supplies service and the competitive
   tendering initiative). There may also be other more localised audit
   findings and criticism that require individual attention (e.g. application of charging regulations for private patients and road traffic
   accident patients).

▼  *Professional inspection*: accreditation for training and other professional requirements are subject to inspection and assessment by a
   variety of professional bodies. In the course of this process, deficiencies in patient or client care are often detected (e.g. beds placed in
   areas not designated for care or treatment – corridors are the cause
   of frequent complaints). These raise important quality considerations which, if prevalent, will again have to be taken into account in
   the business plan.

▼  *Ombudsman and other commissioners*: managers will be concerned
   about the levels of criticism of their record in the execution of statutory and other regulatory obligations with regard to recruitment and
   management of staff, patients and clients. Managers need to follow
   up any complaints and ensure that the correct approach is adopted in
   every case, so that unfortunate incidents are kept to an absolute

minimum. They will want to take steps to eliminate any loopholes that may exist in their employment policy and administration. In all cases managers must make maximum use of conciliatory and mediatory facilities.

▼ *Liability considerations*: as well as being a cost to the organisation, unsettled compensation claims or legal liabilities are indicators of the level of negligence, employer's liability and public liability. Beyond the normal control and disciplinary mechanisms lie the circumstances in which the incidents occurred. Managers need to be acutely aware of these underlying factors and to take steps to see that proper risk assessment and quality control and management procedures are implemented in the future.

▼ *External pressure groups*: these can include a number of vested interests that may or may not find expression through the operation of the local health councils. They often represent important public concerns, and must never be ignored. Often the efforts of groups that are worried about perceived deficiencies in service provision find tangible expression in significant fundraising. This is an area in which relevant managers need to take an interest. As well as being useful future allies, voluntary group efforts can be complementary to funding deficits (*see* Chapter 2).

▼ *Complaints*: although this is part of the bureaucracy of total quality management, verbal complaints made by patients who refuse to articulate their perceptions in writing need to be investigated.

▼ *Legal, ethical and moral pressures*: this modern phenomenon causes dilemmas relating to the appropriateness of care and treatment of certain conditions, and satisfactory protocols need to be agreed.

▼ *Low performance rating*: this is apparent through clinical and other forms of audit, as well as inability to achieve targets.

▼ *Budget deficits*: unless there is an underlying and intractable problem (e.g. relating to funding), a consistent tendency to overspend is an issue that must be addressed in the plan (*see* Chapter 7).

▼ *Security*: poor security record with consistent losses due to both negligence and theft; continual audit criticism and public awareness.

## Checklist of possible opportunities

▼ Developments in clinical practice, new technology and scientific discovery leading to a much broader spectrum of available treatments and care arrangements.

▼ Seed money to assist in the alteration in the balance of care (e.g. a reduction in bed blockers in the acute sector, and children possibly awaiting adoption in care homes in the childcare sector).
▼ Initiatives to improve the management of patient/relative/client expectation and demand and patient/client numbers.
▼ Reallocation of budget savings.
▼ Weaknesses elsewhere.
▼ Opportunities arising from better working practices.
▼ Improvement in a financial growth climate of near zero.
▼ The need to further reduce costs, make savings and increase income.

**Checklist of possible threats**

▼ *Restructuring*: research, reform and increased bureaucracy can result in unsatisfactory quality and wasteful management costs. Demoralisation follows the prospects of changes which may in themselves be uneconomic. Jaded by years of restructuring, the NHS may suffer from an inherent and possibly latent anti-change culture that by inference provides the basis for opposition to anything that smacks of either radicalism or − that fundamental mechanism for change − research.
▼ *Inaccessibility*: the development of and improvement in access to quality healthcare in return for realistic costs are recognisably familiar global problems. As expectations rise, costs tend to have an alarming tendency to escalate in an upward direction. This creates an unstable planning model because there are no evident counterbalancing measures in the equation.
▼ *Confusion*: in the various disparate and sometimes conflicting contexts of the NHS Plan, clinical governance, best value, quality, etc., many organisations within the health and social service spectrum continue to struggle with an integrated approach to the implementation of organisational excellence, performance measurement and process quality improvements.
▼ *Loss of catchment area*: due to competition, general improvement as a result of health education, relocation to improved housing or other social factors can have an impact on a particular specialist ward or unit.
▼ *Beware of retraction models*: an important weapon in the planning arsenal, this can have significant consequences for the long-term future. Unsubstantiated rumours are often as hard to pin down as

they are to deny, so efforts must be directed towards the reduction of turbulence within the organisation. An informed and structured approach needs to be carefully implemented.

▼ *Possible amalgamation with larger unit*: the economic rule that favours economies of scale apparently also tends to pervade the quality of care and treatment insofar as there is a clear lower critical mass below which services are either not safe or not economic (e.g. maternity services in a smaller hospital where deliveries for a rural catchment area may be below acceptable levels and paediatric and neonatal services may therefore not be viable). The loss of these services to a larger unit may well be bad enough for the local population, but there may also be an inherent threat there for other acute services.

▼ *Key staff vacancies*: managers in other disciplines must be constantly aware of the potential threat posed by the prevalence of key staff vacancies to the overall safety and ultimately viability of a multidisciplinary environment.

# Shaping the plan

## Current position

The first step in assessment is to establish a clear picture of the current position. The process may be conveniently broken down into the following components:

- descriptions of current service provisions
- quality initiatives
- analysis of current workloads and dependencies
- resource consumption
- performance levels.

## The historical position

It is important to gain a feel for the traditions of service that have influenced service development so far, when it was founded and for what purpose, and any relevant milestone changes that have occurred along the way. The location and accessibility of the service to the catchment, resident, patch or referred population should also be noted. We can follow this with detailed descriptions of current service provision, volume of care and treatments, size of budget, etc. Particular attention should be paid to service elements that are considered to have star quality (e.g. keyhole surgery, alternative medicine, respite care, etc.).

## Quality initiatives

Arising from the historical notes, valued quality-of-care standards should be noted together with any initiatives that are being used to accurately measure some of the aspirations. For example, the King's Fund accreditation packages, quality circles or total quality management should be included where appropriate.

## Current workloads and dependencies

These must be assessed together with current trends, and need in-depth consideration. However, a number of basic statistics are required:

* the population served
* service capacity
* utilisation or take-up.

## Resource consumption

The implications of supporting current activity levels have to be determined, verified and analysed. This must include staffing, estate, materials, equipment, funding, systems, etc.

## Planning to improve or develop services utilising TOWS results

The next stage in the process is to begin to focus on those areas in both the internal and external environments which have already been identified as threats, opportunities, weaknesses or strengths. It is important to build on positive advantage through the use of main strengths as a starting position. Broad ideas can now be prepared to take advantage of prevailing conditions, so that the best position is achieved in time.

# Operational and action plans

Although planning levels are clearly discernible within an organisation, they are also functions which must be undertaken in smaller collectives, and which the individual must apply to the personal and professional spheres and to the workplace. In the same way, there must be inherent lateral planning which clearly links available resources with service provision. On a comprehensive basis these relationships imbue the various facets of activity with measurable quality.

In complex organisations, the actual bringing together of the plan is a dedicated and identifiable management function, but it must be undertaken at many levels, although they may differ from one another (e.g. providers and commissioners will have slightly different approaches). From the long-term strategy – the *strategic plan* – as events unfold and strategic predictions are tested, it is possible to prepare a shorter plan (usually for a year). This is the *operational plan* (*see* Figure 4.4).

Within this operational plan we can break down the number of management tasks and allocate them to those who will perform them within quite short time scales. This is called the *action plan*.

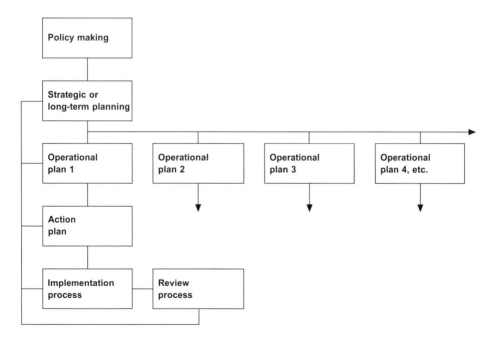

**Figure 4.4**   Operational planning structure.

# Activation

In organisational terms, the activation of a plan at a particular time is critical to both economic mobilisation and relative liquidation of resources appropriate for shorter- and longer-term purposes. It is also important to test the plan and determine whether or not its main purpose is dormant. This is achieved by trying various elements in as realistic a situation as possible. From this, further information must be obtained and further refinements made. Both real and test conditions produce a management loop that enables managers to control activities within the planning process. *Planning and control* are the two management functions that theorists attribute to the administration or bureaucracy associated with a system. Certainly it seems unlikely that the implementation of a plan could succeed without any form of discipline. This is due partly to a lack of co-ordination and partly to the shortage of valid information on how implementation is progressing. The integration of planning and control into a flexible structure requires the arrangement of information in such a way as to facilitate the following:

- implementation − within agreed time scales and at an agreed rate
- monitoring − facilitates the measurement of progress and signal variations
- intervention − at an appropriate time to correct a variable
- revision − takes into account the unexpected
- control − of the overall process.

# Action or roll-out plans

This is the mechanism whereby key tasks, deadlines and responsibilities are agreed. A note of caution should be sounded here. It is not simply a matter of haphazardly handing out jobs to be done so that diaries are nicely filled in and performance review is facilitated. Every task must be treated as a specialist one that requires specific skills and is supported by other members of the management team responsible for that stage. When choosing a manager who is appropriate for the defined task, it is important to bear in mind considerations such as the exposure that the particular role will demand in terms of public and private criticism. Although tasks within the umbrella of business planning may in general be considered to be good for development, other factors (e.g. a prospective manager's status within the organisation, their experience, reputation and credibility, and their emotional resilience) must be given due weight, and consequently some support mechanisms to alleviate the possibility of creating unnecessary stress are essential.

For example, if the stage under consideration is the retraction or reduction of a service, then this can be clearly identified as a distinct event, its completion being determined by a number of characteristics (e.g. no patients/clients, no staff, no heat, light or water, etc.). On the other hand, management development is not a stage but rather an ongoing process that has stages within its compass (e.g. the management of a specific course).

---

**Tips from the front office**

▼ Although data, statistics, graphs and relevant facts, are the fundamental tools that facilitate plan construction, they should be assembled at the back of the working plan.

▼ Don't include irrelevant or out-of-date data to bulk out the document.

▼ To save time later, write up all the background descriptions, sense of vision for the future, and sustainable quality objectives – put these into the plan format and have them ready for the final document.

▼ Working forward, the main body of the plan should also contain the guiding principles, the options, the argument and the main conclusions.

▼ A management summary should be included at the front of the document.

▼ Thus, the substance of the plan can be as in Figure 4.5.

---

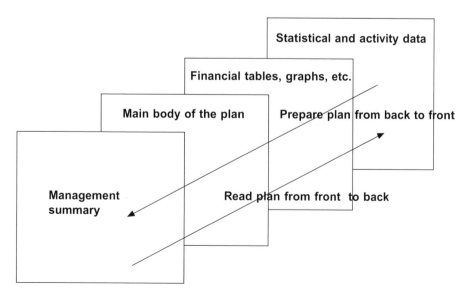

**Figure 4.5**   Business plan construction.

# Case study

Examples of some of the process quality issues included in the joint Near-Home Facility Plan are listed below.

## Transport services

- Development of protocols for the acceptance of requests for urgent and non-urgent transport services.

## Acute services

- Further development of protocols for discharge of bed blockers to the Near-Home joint facility.
- Extension of day procedures, with due regard for appropriateness, recovery time needed, fitness for discharge and domestic circumstances.
- Selected pilot-scheme protocols for the introduction and evaluation of pathways of care, including work with Near-Home facility staff.

## Care of the elderly

- Development of differentiated response protocols that reflect the needs of care management and take into account the greatly increased levels of demand.
- Implementation of compliance protocols for health and safety, fire precautions, control of *Legionella*, and building and electrical regulations.

## Rehabilitation

- Protocols relating to the reshaping of health and social care to achieve a better balance between obtaining greater independence for patients and clients and the cost of service delivery.

## Security

- Upgrading systems, additional staffing and equipment.

# 5

# Influencing the supply chain

Although they are probably unaware of their passive influence, all managers and staff are at the centre of resource consumption. They may only notice when an expected event, such as the delivery of necessary materials or the arrival of a new recruit, fails to occur. A sudden surge in budget expenditure may momentarily grab their attention, but perhaps other more pressing tasks quickly distract them. Without much deeper thought they may be willing to accept compromises or dubious explanations for unsatisfactory goods and services. In the longer term, their possible indifference to or ignorance of the significance of the so-called *supply chain* can be severely detrimental to acceptable practice, and may be a potential threat to patient/client safety.

In order to perform their various different tasks efficiently and effectively, managers need to have essential resources when these are required. From the organisation's point of view, these resources must be obtained at the best value for money. Therefore the supply chain is dedicated to obtaining the following:

- goods and services of the right *quality*
- in the right *quantities*
- at the right *time*
- in the right *place*
- for the right *price*.

However, this process must be subjected to user scrutiny and approval so that the overall objectives are achieved. Managers and frontline staff must participate in and influence the supply chain so that waste and costs are minimised and the best possible goods and services are thus obtained.

## The issues

The estimated value of the health and social care estate is £33 billion, and the day-to-day cost of running the service is estimated to be around £66 billion, of which 70–80% is spent on personnel. Although the management and control of payroll costs are absorbing and at times sophisticated, experience indicates that the smaller 20–30% segment of expenditure on estate, equipment, materials, etc. provides a greater challenge. This is due to a number of factors – mainly the disparate nature of these elements together with the multitude of demand sources and difficulties in maintaining control of the cost of individual items. However, the frontline user manager can have a major beneficial influence.

---

**Checklist of key frontline user supply line relationships**

The frontline user has key relationships with the following:

▼    the purchasing organisation or manager who is responsible for the specialist contracting process. These relationships are usually limited to:
  – personnel for human resources (70–80% of running costs)
  – pharmacy for drugs, etc.
  – estate services for building, grounds and engineering
  – catering manager or contractor for provisions, etc.
  – contracts manager for goods and services that have been contracted out
  – supplies organisation for most other goods and services
▼    the external service provider or supplier who, through a process of market testing (or in the case of personnel, application and interview), has been selected as the most competent and competitive
▼    the paymaster, who must be satisfied that the resources were required in the first instance, and were properly received subject to contract conditions, before payment is made.

---

These relationships are illustrated in Figure 5.1.

As well as the benefits derived from specialisation, this organisational division of main tasks ensures the integrity of the paymaster system. However, there is a need for good communications in the user/purchaser/paymaster triangle. In addition, a balance must be struck between the separation of powers and duties within the structure. In order to maximise the benefits, most organisations try to maintain a degree of independence between function and lines of professional responsibility.

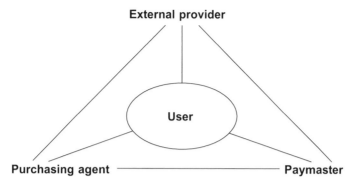

**Figure 5.1**   User/purchaser/paymaster structure and division.

| Function | Responsibility |
| --- | --- |
| Expression of need | Frontline user/manager |
| Authority to purchase | Supplies/personnel/pharmacist/estate/etc. |
| Identification of budget | Frontline user/manager/finance |
| Contracting and purchasing | Supplies/personnel/pharmacist/estate, etc. and frontline user/manager |
| Delivery | As appropriate (e.g. stores personnel) |
| Receipt | Frontline user/manager |
| Method of payment | Paymaster staff |
| Method of accountancy | Accounting staff |
| Audit | Absolute independence |

The outside supplier should be excluded from all of these detailed activities except where regulations require participation (e.g. tendering, negotiation and contracting obligations).

---

**Tips from the front office**

▼    The number of managers who have authority to enter contracts and place orders must be restricted. The manager who signs the contract or order must not be made responsible for paying the bills. This is difficult in smaller organisations (e.g. in the voluntary sector) or where fundraising events are being planned.

Frontline users and managers therefore have a crucial influence on the efficiency and effectiveness of resource purchasing. Whether or not they are aware of it, this places a burden of responsibility upon them to obtain the quality and quantity of resources needed to enable them to perform their disparate tasks.

# Influencing the supply chain

The chain of events that arises from any one or a number of purchasing requirements is usually referred to as the *supply chain*. However, this does not conform to an annual time-frame. For example, it can be protracted where new buildings are constructed or, in the case of a run-of-the-mill item, it might be achieved almost immediately, depending on supply. The supply chain describes those events which characterise the way in which an item is requested, purchased, received, distributed, paid for and accounted for. It includes all resources (i.e. personnel, estate, equipment, materials, etc.).

Figure 5.2 illustrates the supply chain that is used for the purchase of most goods and services. Other resources, such as personnel, are obtained according to the same broad principles, but clearly differ in some respects.

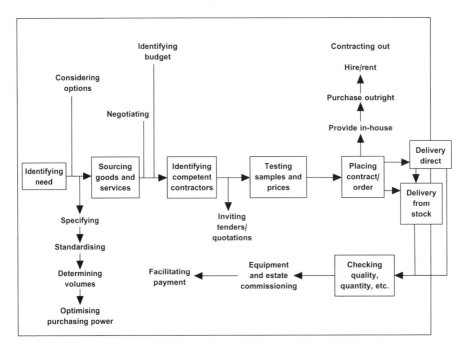

**Figure 5.2** The supply chain.

Partly as a consequence of the smooth running of the system, and partly due to the pressure under which managers and frontline staff have to work, waste and losses to the organisation may occur because of inattention to detail.

**Checklist of key points at which waste or loss may occur**

▼ *Requirement*: the stipulated requirement may be unnecessary, incorrectly described or inappropriate, or there might be a suitable alternative. If the request is processed, the item purchased will in the short or medium term become obsolete, and time and money will be wasted.

**Tips from the front office**

▼ Be sure of your facts.
▼ Do not allow yourself to be bullied into accepting a cheaper alternative.
▼ Get involved in order to get what you really need.

▼ *Volumes*: if more than one item is needed, estimating the correct volume is crucial to purchasing at the best price from a contractor who is competent to provide that level of service because of the expected economies of scale. When frontline users order quantities in excess of their reasonable requirements, this only leads to stockpiling in inappropriate places and wastage through loss, pilfering or expiry of shelf-life.

**Tips from the front office**

▼ Check out your ordering and reordering arrangements.
▼ Reduce levels where appropriate.
▼ Look out for stock or redundant equipment that is taking up otherwise valuable space, and have them written off.

▼ *Level of purchasing*: this is decided partly by the type of proposed purchase, partly by the expected volumes and partly the scale of the purchase. For example, a single small item that is not kept in store may be purchased from petty cash, whereas a large number of low-cost items may be subjected to a full-scale purchasing procedure and may in future be retained in stores. However, single items that have a high price tag, such as certain items of medical equipment, may require specialist purchasing arrangements and consequently the process may take time to complete. Losses of time, effort and money can occur as a result of either purchasing at an inappropriate level or a lack of frontline user appreciation of the time scales involved.

---

**Tips from the front office**

▼   Order larger items early and with precision in order to avoid disappointment.

---

▼   *Standardising*: the compulsion to standardise arises from a desire for interchangeability, the potential exercise of purchasing power, a general lowering of stock levels and an overall improvement in efficiency. If there is an important reason for your request not to be subjected to these criteria, make sure that you have the details to hand (e.g. clinical preference, or the contrary results of recent trials).

▼   *Sourcing*: the main supply sources may already be well known, but you may know of others that should be tested (e.g. professional journals or newspapers in other languages where job vacancies could be advertised). It may also be that at this stage a decision is necessary as to whether to contract out particular elements, hire or rent them, or provide them in-house (e.g. sterile fluids and sterile supplies, or stationery that can be computer generated).

▼   *Selecting competent contractors*: the judgement here hinges upon such matters as the following:
    − reputation and reliability as a provider
    − ability to handle the volumes required
    − employment policies that are compatible with health and social care organisations.

▼   *Quotation/tendering procedures*: in the case of smaller one-off items contractors already tested may be asked to provide a quotation. Where larger-scale purchasing is required, although for reasons already covered, the lowest tender may not be successful, secure tendering arrangements are necessary. This usually means that tenders must be received by a certain date and time, and kept securely under lock and key by an independent party who, together with a second independent person, opens them, records the contents and submits the results to a designated manager for appropriate action.

▼ *Testing samples*: as part of the tendering procedure, samples may be submitted, and here the frontline user/manager must be a willing participant of the testing/validating process. Membership of materials user forums (MUFs) dedicated to testing and standardising is also important. Although it is not so obvious, the potential for waste at this juncture occurs in cases where purchases are simply not fit for the job.

---

**Tips from the front office**

▼   Make sure that you treat the sampling process seriously.
▼   Listen to the experiences of both supplies experts and colleagues.

---

▼ *Placing a contract/order*: time, energy and money can be wasted if a contract or order is inappropriately placed.

---

**Tips from the front office**

▼   Be aware of the correct sources of supply.

---

▼ *Stock items*: in order to reduce repetitive ordering and ensure a constant supply of small to medium cost and size items, reasonable supplies should be kept in secure stores which are located either on site or at a central location that is convenient to as large a number of users as possible. Stocks at this level are under constant review to ensure that they do not go out of date or that for one reason or another demand is about to decrease or cease altogether. Arrangements for supply to wards, departments and units vary. Sometimes supply is in response to a requisition, and sometimes it involves automatic items arriving 'just in time' (JIT) or alternatively items may be delivered on a 'topping up' basis. In all cases, frontline staff and managers must ensure that stockpiling (which results in waste, obsolescence, pilfering, etc.) does not occur, and that deliveries are correct and are really required.

---

**Tips from the front office**

▼   Where a change in policy is contemplated (e.g. uniforms, stationery, laundry items), make sure that adequate notice is

> given so that centrally held stocks can be reduced or at least not reordered. It is not sufficient to assume that this will happen automatically.

▼ *Accepting and delivery*: always make sure that the goods are delivered in good condition, in the correct quantities, and that the quality is of the standard required. This is a good defence against pilfering.

**Tips from the front office**

▼ If there is a problem, make sure that both the supplies department and the accounts department are made aware of this, preferably in writing, so that proper action is taken at the correct time.

▼ *Commissioning equipment, etc.*: new equipment and estate should be subject to an agreed commissioning procedure, which may involve the correct unpacking of equipment and its demonstration by an expert. Failure to ensure that this is properly supervised and executed can result in breakages or malfunctioning.

▼ *Facilitating payment*: when all the relevant parts of the transaction have been properly completed, ensure that documentation is signed and dispatched to facilitate payment. Failure to do this not only causes frustration and wastes time, but can also result in the loss of discounts for prompt settlement or even the breach of contract conditions and the suspension of supply. Complications arise from the cost of the length of the supply chain. If the chain is short, there is only a small time lapse between the expression of need and receipt. In these circumstances, price variations and other deviations (e.g. possible loss of discount) are unlikely to occur. If the supply chain is longer, significant differences may occur between the amount approved and the amount that is finally paid out.

Resources flow in many directions throughout an organisation, and range from stationery for the front office to essential ingredients for the shop floor. It is crucial to the success of an organisation that supply and distribution processes which secure the right quantity and quality at the right price are maintained without the need to stockpile. Unfortunately, regardless of size and scope, active participation in these arrangements and the release of appropriate regulatory documentation are not seen as priorities by departmental managers.

Below is a checklist of basic essential activities and a list of tips.

---

**Checklist of dos and don'ts**

Remember that these matters affect your budget performance.

*Do*

▼   Participate in all materials user forums (MUFs) aimed at standardising specifications and obtaining value for money (VFM).
▼   Encourage creativity in supply chain management and note any complaints from operatives.
▼   Facilitate new product trials and comment positively – engage properly with product evaluation teams (PETs).
▼   Contribute to the pre- and post-contract negotiating process.
▼   Generate order communications in accordance with agreed time scales and methodologies.
▼   Check the quality and quantity of all goods received immediately.
▼   Notify immediately any doubts about contractor compliance.
▼   Clear all queries and documentation without delay.
▼   Contribute fully to review processes.

*Don't*

▼   Waste time and energy on hostility to supply chain initiatives whose objectives are unattractive.
▼   Economise at the expense of health and safety.
▼   Ignore complaints or warnings about potential hazards.
▼   Take unnecessary risks.
▼   Stockpile – instead, keep stocks to a minimum. Over-stocking leads to temptation to pilfer, and is also costly to maintain.
▼   Allow materials to become out of date.

---

**Tips from the front office**

▼   Quality is compliance with the appropriate specification – it is *not* usually the most expensive item.

▼ Quantities should always be exact – make sure that you are using the correct unit (i.e. one only, tens, dozens, hundreds, gross, etc.).
▼ Check out the efficacy of just-in-time (JIT) stock management systems.
▼ Where stocks are maintained at low levels, timely deliveries are essential.

# Supply chain contingency management

In the modern peacetime world of commerce, until recently no threat to or interruption of supplies has been perceived, and lines are often tortuously long. Stores and stockpiling are still regarded as wasteful, and there is heavy reliance on just-in-time deliveries. However, the recent petrol delivery crisis, when a standstill was imminent after only a few days, together with the realisation following the foot-and-mouth crisis that food in all its forms is often transported over incredible distances to reach the consumer, have made the Government and managers think again about reserves. Below is a check-list of basic links in the supply chain where planned contingencies may be inserted and controlled, together with tips.

**Checklist of intervention points**

▼ *User requirements, sourcing supplies and specifications*:
  – examine volumes and move towards appropriate standardisation
  – simplify and rationalise the number of similar items in specifications.
▼ *Evaluate purchasing power and identify strategic alliances*: examine the options for increasing purchasing power through partnership or agency arrangements with other purchasing organisations.
▼ *Develop corporate policy on contingency requirements*:
  – ensure flexibility in contract arrangements
  – delegate more purchasing to local level
  – look at vertical integration and just-in-time policies.
▼ *Choose competent contractors*: by established reputation, these contractors can guarantee supplies. Check out the nature of these assurances.
▼ *Post-tender negotiations*: it is sometimes considered appropriate to follow up the receipt of tenders with briefing or debriefing sessions when both further considerations and more details are discussed and agreed. These can include concerns over deliveries.

▼ *Review facilities*: for the reception and storage of goods and services and secure adequate provision.
▼ *Constantly review*: contingency reserves through adequate audit and other systems.

---

**Tips from the front office**

▼ Quality in terms of volume can often be obtained at an agreed cost.
▼ Limited volume can mask under-utilised resources.
▼ Low volumes can be a threat to safety, due to lack of practice.
▼ High volumes may also be unsafe because of overwork.
▼ Plan for only adequate contingencies.
▼ Ensure that contingency shelf-lives are appropriate.
▼ Contingency movements should comply with usual first-in, first-out arrangements.

# Payroll and the culture of competence

From the earliest times, morale has generally been recognised to be one of the key factors that facilitates or reduces an organisation's capacity to be successful. The ability to recognise and improve poor or low morale is therefore an essential management attribute, and taking proper measures will enhance performance. In health and social care organisations, the budget for staff can represent 80% of the total revenue budget. Below is a checklist of some basic general management principles that will encourage improvements in performance and reduce waste.

---

**Checklist of improvements**

▼ *Get to know your staff*:
   – become involved in recruitment and induction of your own staff
   – ensure that your training programme is appropriate to each level of skill
   – get involved in the induction processes of other disciplines
   – make sure that you know your own staff on a personal basis.
▼ *Establish a performance database*: this database should include sickness, absenteeism, accidents, complaints, negligence, mistakes, fraud,

deliberate vandalism, etc. and any other untoward events. Obtain comparisons from similar departments and/or other organisations, keep records of disciplinary matters, and assess the state of morale based on reliable data.

▼ *Clear and achievable objectives*: conflicting or (taking account of resource levels) impossible objectives decrease morale. Ensure that there is a sense of direction, give and obtain commitment, and re-member that agreed mission statements are often efficacious.

▼ *Discipline*: make sure that the organisation's code of conduct is reason-able, appropriate and acceptable, and that it is applied impartially.

▼ *Departmental/unit pride and profile*:
  – generate pride through teamworking
  – provide team figures for productivity and market share
  – encourage ideas for general improvement
  – support developments that will lead to expansion of the patient/client base.

▼ *Structure and organisation*:
  – where appropriate, divide and apportion workloads to specialist teams
  – structure teams to reflect defined responsibilities
  – make sure that the numbers on your budget agree with the actual numbers of staff who are working in your department.

▼ *Behaviour and equality*:
  – promote and accept only the highest standards of behaviour
  – develop and foster an atmosphere of mutual respect
  – ensure that maximum privacy and confidentiality are accorded to all
  – personally deal with all complaints and criticisms, and be quietly persistent
  – ensure that all employees are treated with equal respect
  – ensure that all employees are paid according to the work they do, not according to who or what they are
  – take steps to correct deficiency, and keep it under review.

▼ *Conditions of employment*: as well as rewards and remuneration, con-ditions can be systematically improved by enhancing the working environment so that it is appropriate to the tasks undertaken. Health and safety, cleanliness, lighting, heat, decoration, state of repair, and canteen and toilet facilities are simple considerations that all affect workforce morale.

▼ *Awkward patient/client relationships*: high patient/client expectations coupled with the frustration of dealing with a large and apparently impersonal organisation have in recent years produced the phenom-enon of customer rage. Staff who have to deal with such problems may experience lowered morale, and management must take a pro-active role in providing support.

▼ *Rewarding competence*:
  – standardise and rate methodologies that are appropriate to each payroll task
  – develop specialist skill levels and integrate them with appropriate qualifications
  – reward staff commensurately according to workload demands
  – do not confuse excessive speed with efficiency and effectiveness
  – prepare succession plans.

▼ *Training*:
  – induction and ongoing training programmes are important assets
  – make sure that feelings and complaints expressed in the classroom are properly channelled into the system so that their impact can be assessed
  – utilise the workplace as a management college for teams and individuals.

▼ *Communication*: an open system of communications and information will help to dispel any adverse rumours or, at worst, will facilitate the management of bad news.

---

**Tips from the front office**

▼ A plan based on a survey of the above factors converted into acceptability criteria can be readily drawn up, but its implementa-tion needs to be measured against both databases and observations, so that a genuine rise in morale is seen to be matched by improve-ments in productivity and a reduction in waste.

---

# Achieving payroll accuracy

Staff who consistently receive pay that is incorrect, or who receive their pay at the wrong time, or receive no pay at all, are not going to be part of a happy and highly motivated workforce. In addition, these inaccuracies will be reflected in budget statements, and will cause unexpected fluctuations. It will therefore be difficult to predict future trends. Frontline staff and managers must find and eradicate the causes of payroll problems.

It is easy to blame payroll staff for such inaccuracies, but frequently the faults lie elsewhere because the correct information has not been properly conveyed to the point of payment. This damages an important interdependency, especially where a manager has failed to comply with deadlines. These include the payment of new recruits, promotions, exceptions and irregular features such as overtime, special duty payments and other changes in circumstances. Co-operation rather than deadlock through agreed protocols is essential.

Below is a checklist of relevant considerations.

---

**Checklist of payroll protocols**

▼   *Payroll systems*:
   − where deficiencies have been detected as a result of staff complaint, audit, review or other techniques, managers need to be amenable to any necessary investigation
   − they need to understand significant factors and to co-operate
   − communication can be improved by networking with key departmental heads
   − computerisation should reduce drudgery but not replace intelligence
   − be aware of system security weaknesses.
▼   *Documentation flows*:
   − maintain the flow of necessary documentation
   − utilise remote data-capture techniques wherever possible
   − protect audit trails and introduce efficient tracking systems
   − communications relating to budgetary, costing, statistical or other performance indicators must be made part of an ongoing dialogue
   − new performance initiatives should be agreed with heads of departments before commencement.
▼   *Lines and modes of communication*:
   − responsibilities and authorities must be defined for accountability purposes
   − rather than forcing every issue to the top of the office, realistic contact points for routine dialogue should be established further down the hierarchical chain
   − finance managers need to convince other heads that their role is always a helpful one.

---

**Tips from the front office**

▼   Keep relationships with heads of other departments on a professional basis.
▼   Make sure that all of your data and other facts are accurate before you engage in communication. Ask more than once 'Can this be right?', and check it again! Failure can damage your credibility.
▼   Never create the impression that you are in competition for points.

# Case study

Ms Nora Rightly consistently failed to meet deadlines for the enrolment of new staff and the submission of overtime sheets. This resulted in an apparently significant underspending on her payroll budget. Around the same time she also refused to accept some of the furniture which had been ordered as part of the Near-Home facility refurbishment scheme. The reason for her refusal was that two of the items had been slightly damaged by the carrier.

Eventually she was persuaded to take the whole delivery into safekeeping on the understanding that the matter would be satisfactorily resolved. Until that time, Ms Rightly would not sign that she had received the articles. Unfortunately, no one informed the finance department, and in addition to losing the 5% settlement discount (around £1000), her goods and services budget was showing an underspending of £20 000 at the end of the financial period.

Apparently, being unaware of all the details, Midas Luckpenny was pleased to be able to report the cumulative good fortune to the management team.

After the meeting, Ms Rightly wanted to know why Midas Luckpenny had not reported the loss, as she was expecting a reprimand. He put his finger over his lips in a gesture of confidentiality, but Nora Rightly suspected that he had something more to hide. Her suspicions were confirmed when she received her budget statement the following month, which showed the extra payments – but the budget target had also been adjusted upward.

# 6

# Making a bid for additional resources

Frontline managers, those who have recently become budget managers, and those who have considerable experience of budget management are always keen to develop and improve the service that they provide. However, they are often perplexed when their bid for additional resources is unsuccessful. There are many reasons for this failure. Sometimes it is impossible for individual managers to discover the weaknesses of their cases, but answering the question 'Did you do the right thing, first time, every time?' is a good way to gather at least a few clues.

Although it seems an obvious negative judgement criterion, seeking funds for a project that is completely contrary to the strategic objectives of an organisation will have no chance of success. Similarly, a proposal that is too vast in terms of time or money is unlikely to succeed in that form. And even small bids at a time when there are simply no funds available for development have a doubtful outcome unless the manager can identify financial and other benefits that will cancel the initial expenditure.

This chapter aims to provide a structure for managers who are preparing a case – perhaps for the first time. It gives guidance on the elements that will be of benefit and those that reduce the prospects of success. After reading this chapter you will:

- understand the likely financial rules and their impact
- be able to list demands in a logical fashion
- have an understanding of how to prioritise internal demands
- know when and how to reassess priorities during a financial period.

## The issues

Successful bids for additional resources must conform both to the overall strategic objectives of the organisation and to the broadly based development or improvement plans mentioned in Chapter 4. To recapitulate, the key external environmental pressures that may produce additional funds arise from an improved official awareness of the following:

- an increasingly dependent elderly population
- a growing demand for specialist services
- the pressures of a general escalation of patient/client numbers
- increased patient/relative/client expectations
- financial pressures arising from legal, ethical and moral judgements.

In the context of this awareness of external pressures, the checklist below shows the internal developments or improvements that are most likely to attract additional funding.

---

**Checklist of internal developments or improvements**

▼   Graded bids to develop or improve the internal physical environment – improving the condition or quality of the estate, equipment, fabric or furniture.

▼   Bids based on developments or improvements that lead to a much broader spectrum of available treatments and care arrangements – funds required for staff and/or equipment.

▼   Local initiatives that provide increasing support and care for an ageing population – short-term limited additional funds may be available for creative ideas.

▼   Unacceptable waiting times and length of waiting lists, including the length of time that patients/clients have to spend in waiting areas.

▼   Continued change in the balance of care in favour of care in the community (e.g. bed blockers in the acute sector, and children possibly awaiting adoption in care homes in the childcare sector).

---

In a financial growth climate of near zero, there is a constant need to further reduce costs, make savings and increase income. Innovative schemes that conform with some of the criteria set out above have a significantly better chance of success, provided that they meet certain financial criteria. Below is a checklist of the main financial considerations.

---

**Checklist of financial criteria that improve a bid's chance of success**

▼   Bids that guarantee a measure of financial improvement.

▼   Bids that include an element of self-finance.

▼ Bids that offer improvement through a partnership with a suitable organisation.

Other financial considerations that may influence the success of a bid include the following.

▼ The reputation of the author as a prudent and thrifty manager (*see* Chapter 7).
▼ The size and scope of the proposal (don't get carried away – keep bids in proportion).
▼ The relative time scales involved – make sure that deliveries can be achieved within the time scales laid down (i.e. usually before the end of the current financial year).
▼ The expected consumption patterns.

In the long run, funding is dependent on a system of priorities, and managers must prioritise competing demands in order to bid successfully.

▼ Funds that are made available for one specific purchase means that delivery must be accomplished within the allocated time-frame.
▼ In contrast, repetitive expenditure (e.g. payroll) will usually be funded over a longer time-frame.

# Listing demands

When listing developments that will greatly enhance the performance of their departments, managers often forget that if their existing resources are in poor condition or their working life is close to termination, these mundane demands must also be taken into account.

In addition, when considering the general planning criteria mentioned above, you should also ensure that you have a comprehensive list of other demands.

When assessing future demands on available resources, an indication of the impact of their condition is essential to their utility.

Below are two checklists that are relevant to these considerations.

**Checklist of general considerations with regard to the internal environment**

▼ Conduct an assessment of available resources (time, estate, equipment, expertise, expendibles, etc.).

▼ Give consideration to your historical legacy (past performance, goodwill, etc.).

▼ Take account of how your organisation/unit measures up to present standards.

▼ Make sure that you have covered all aspects of development:
  − technical
  − environmental.

▼ Perform an analysis of your existing level of funding (*see* Chapter 7).

---

**Checklist of condition of resources**

▼ The expected working life of all assets, including labour, should be tested against maintenance costs and a timetable of replacement needs.

▼ The lifespan of items, goods, services and materials can be fairly accurately assessed, and although it usually has long-term implications, payroll also has obvious and known working-life implications.

▼ This lifespan inventory can be reviewed in the light of current developments, repairs, sickness, etc., to see whether obsolescence is more inherent.

▼ Possible replacement problems should be considered in the light of opportunity, alternatives and the potential contribution of the item to the general care plan.

▼ If it is decided to confirm the asset review findings and to process a firm proposal, there should be a clearly defined financial benefit.

▼ Day-to-day items such as withdrawals from stockpiles or stores and ongoing payroll would not usually be the subject of this type of review, which is intended to apply only to marginal activity where impending obsolescence is detected.

▼ When the need has been identified, interested parties consulted and a proposal framed, further progress can only be made against a background of agreed policy.

▼ This usually means that, due to limited funds, some low-priority items on the shopping list will not be processed, but will be kept pending further developments.

▼ Make sure that all items are costed at the best possible price.

▼ If possible, divide larger amounts into component parts. If large items are all part of one package, you should consider a separate funding bid.

# Prioritising competing demands

Much has been written about budgeting, rationing and prioritisation. They are emotive subjects, but in reality all successful managers in whatever activity they choose have learned to match the appropriate amount of resources – from a lamentably scarce supply – to meet escalating and increasingly excessive demands.

*This skill is a key management competence, and it is important that frontline managers become familiar with the relevant mechanisms, rather than depending on instinct alone.*

In the context of health and social care, a potentially successful bid must fit within a selected limited number of competing dependencies. It is a matter of identifying the correct priorities. In a simple situation, there are a number of ways in which to categorise resource demands.

Below is a series of checklists that will help you to develop this competence.

---

**Checklist of first steps**

1   Take the comprehensive list of realistic proposals (say A, B, C, D, E, F).
2   Set out key criteria. For example:
   ▼   health and safety issues
   ▼   conformity with the overall direction
   ▼   cost of the proposal
   ▼   savings, if any
   ▼   benefits, including intangible ones.
3   Under each criterion give a rating (say from one to five).
4   Add across and put demands in priority order according to the rating (*see* Table 6.1).

---

**Table 6.1**   Prioritising competing demands

| Item | Safety | Direction | Cost | Savings | Benefits | Score | Rank |
|------|--------|-----------|------|---------|----------|-------|------|
| A | 5 | 3 | 2 | 1 | 3 | 14 | 3 |
| B | 4 | 2 | 3 | 5 | 2 | 16 | 1 |
| C | 3 | | 4 | | | 7 | 6 |
| D | 2 | 1 | | 3 | 5 | 11 | 4 |
| E | 1 | 5 | 1 | 4 | 4 | 15 | 2 |
| F | | 4 | 5 | 2 | 1 | 12 | 5 |
| Total | 15 | 15 | 15 | 15 | 15 | 75 | |

In this example the priority order is B, E, A, D, F, C. However, it must be remembered that the method of scoring must be made appropriate to your needs.

The imposition of artificial time limits (e.g. the end of the financial year) has important consequences for priority ratings when decisions are being taken about future spending. The above example takes no account of timing for the task or service required. If some of the items or tasks could not be delivered in time, it would be pointless considering them until their delivery could be assured within the required time scale. Thus, for example, if items B and E could not be delivered, the priorities would have to be changed as follows.

| Item | Old rank | Old score | Multiply by time | New score | New rank | Comments |
|------|----------|-----------|------------------|-----------|----------|----------|
| A | 3 | 14 | 1 | 14 | 1 | |
| B | 1 | 16 | Zero | Zero | – | Add to next period? |
| C | 6 | 7 | 1 | 7 | 4 | |
| D | 4 | 11 | 1 | 11 | 3 | |
| E | 2 | 15 | Zero | Zero | – | Add to next period? |
| F | 5 | 12 | 1 | 12 | 2 | |
| Total | – | 75 | – | – | – | |

# Reassessing priorities during a financial period

It sometimes happens that circumstances change during a financial year. For example:

- deadlines cannot be met
- delays occur with delivery dates
- predicted savings can or cannot be achieved to a greater or lesser extent
- additional funds can or cannot be made available
- an unexpected crisis with existing resources occurs.

Therefore it is important to be able to reassess your list of priorities quickly.

With an expiring time limit (e.g. nearing the end of a financial year) there is a temptation to expedite a purchase or to offer a modest alternative because of a lack of funds. Expediency would never be viewed as an efficient device,

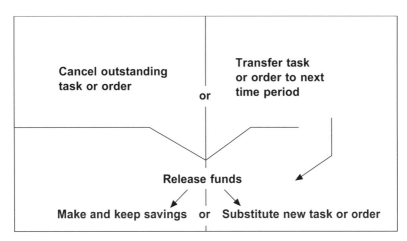

**Figure 6.1**    The exchange dilemma.

and for this reason most organisations ensure that some kind of administrative machinery is available to frustrate potentially wasteful endeavours.

This in turn creates a dilemma in the response to urgency, which is tempered by natural caution (*see* Figure 6.1).

However, the main distinguishing feature depends on the resolution of the expediency/caution dilemma. The 'expedient' situation, where the consultative machinery has been partially adopted or totally ignored, can only result in dissatisfaction and is the acid test of quality. During the early stages, system changes would be necessary in order to eliminate the possibility that either too much frustration is caused due to cumbersome systems based on a cautionary approach, or too much dissatisfaction arises from the expedient approach.

Identification of a genuine opportunity that will enable an organisation to dispose of funds within the limits is a measure of its progressive image. In satisfying management's acquisitive nature, inherent in the tendency towards organised purchase, therefore, there should be no apparent loss of momentum, yet the sequence of events may envisage a fairly long purchasing and commissioning process.

Speed in decision taking is inhibited both by good purchasing practice and by the need to consult. On the other hand, in making good use of a range of expertise in the corporate context, the logical progression of events may be so organised that needs and opportunities are graded such that a scale of priorities is established prior to the budgetary period.

The main emphasis is on keeping tasks and cost below the target line during the agreed period. This is achieved by constantly reviewing the outstanding priorities. At key intervals these are reduced by those items which will not come to fruition during the period and introducing others which are not subject to the same delay.

---

**Tips from the front office**

▼  With the expiry of the time limit, the expenditure will tend to equal the budget, and the model within defined time limits would be the relationship which exists between target, commitment, supply chain and the final completed work.

---

# Bridging the funding gap

A bid for additional resources is more likely to succeed if the frontline manager identifies the source(s) from which funds may become available. These may include a wide spectrum of sources (e.g. new monies, savings, additional income, free funds, etc.).

Below is a checklist of possible funding sources, with details of availability criteria.

---

**Checklist of possible funding sources**

▼  *New money*:
  – Government initiatives, such as the waiting-list initiative
  – development that has already been agreed.
▼  *Savings*:
  – from alteration in the balance of care, resulting in reallocation
  – from reuse of redundant building stock, heating, maintenance
  – from increased efficiency
  – budget savings.
▼  *Increased income*:
  – from increased use of facilities
  – from payments from patients and clients
  – from contributions from other sources.
▼  *Partnerships*: with other statutory agencies and legitimate commercial concerns.
▼  *Free funds*: use of specific funds for legitimate purposes.
▼  *Friends groups*: support from organisations dedicated to raising funds for a specific purpose (e.g. cardiac care associations may partially support the purchase of specific equipment for cardiac care).

# Case study

The Near-Home development team reported on the likely savings to be made from further initiatives to reduce the number of patients in the acute sector who were 'blocking beds' together with other funds that would support the Near-Home initiative.

Their calculations were the result of a detailed study, an outline of which is shown below.

| Detail | Amount (£) |
|---|---|
| Waiting-list initiative | 250 000 |
| Social Services joint funding contribution | 200 000 |
| Savings from redundant building stock, etc. | 50 000 |
| Income from residents | 250 000 |
| Total full year cost | 750 000 |

There would also be a saving of an unidentified amount of capital monies held in reserve.

On the developmental side, bids for additional funding to support the balance of care initiative were still being considered, but initial estimates were as follows.

- Revenue cost of client care – £510 000.
- Revenue cost of rehabilitation facilities (daily living, etc.) – £110 000.
- Additional revenue costs of a multidisciplinary pathway of care team for individual assessment and care management to cover the short-, medium- and longer-term needs, including acute care and aftercare – £55 000.
- Additional cost of comprehensive rehabilitation and follow-up pro- grammes to enable individuals to make the transition towards greater independence – £42 000.
- Additional cost of arrangements for management development, monitor- ing, review and evaluation of programmes – £40 000.

*Total revenue estimate: £757 000.*

- Capital cost of refurbishing and commissioning a 'new' facility to accom- modate the assessment and rehabilitation unit, and to include respite day centre – £500 000.

# 7

# Making the most of budget management systems

The prevalence of money shortages has always been a daunting phenomenon, but it is one that effective budgetary management aims to minimise.

Nevertheless, both first-time frontline managers and more experienced managers often find the objectives of an organisation's budget management system confusing and frustrating.

Unfortunately, defects in the management arrangements may militate against effective management. This chapter looks at potential difficulties and provides managers at all levels with remedial guidance relating to the following:

- the importance of good two-way communication
- the impact of resource mobility
- structural limitations
- restricted delegation and the viability of budgets
- the relationship between workload, dependency, cost and budget.

## The issues

A budget is an allocation of money or a ration of resources (e.g. people) intended for a specific purpose and limited by time (e.g. a week, a month or a year). Nowadays, most budgets are expressed in money terms, but they often incorporate supporting data which show the items that could be purchased or that have been purchased.

For simplicity, budgets can be divided into two basic types. Those which occur frequently and almost equally (e.g. basic payroll) are called *regularly occurring budgets*. Budgets that are intended for infrequent spending (e.g. equipment, works, some forms of payroll, etc.) are called *non-recurring budgets*.

However, there are many variations in different systems, attitudes and applications. Most simple budgets are based on the areas managed by key professionals. Usually they are easily identified:

- by location (a ward, department or unit), *or*
- by discipline or profession (e.g. medical, nursing, social services, administration), *or*
- by speciality firm (e.g. general surgery, medicine, paediatrics, etc.), *or*
- by some combination that is unique to and suitable for a particular situation.

The amount and level of funding are issues that need to be clearly understood. Budgets must reflect the following:

- the amount of resources to be purchased
- the agreed quality of service to be performed
- the expected workloads relating to levels of dependency
- the overall costs ratios at certain levels of performance.

In order to develop a budget management system, communication is essential. The assembly of facts and figures must both capture the initialisation and convey the need to take action. Skills in managing within the budgetary environment must also be developed. Enhanced interpretative and intervention capacity is key to improved performance. Clarity, timing, focus, action and reaction are the objectives of good communication.

---

**Checklist of budget system communication characteristics**

▼ *Accuracy*:
  - complete and transparent reconciliation of facts and figures
  - amendments are unnecessary
  - variations at each stage must be identified.
▼ *Simplicity*:
  - format is easily read and understood
  - clear statement of financial objectives
  - no unnecessary detail is included
  - familiarity with terminology.
▼ *Timeliness*:
  - financial information is available to budget managers in time for them to take remedial action

  - a reduction in potential losses as a result of prompt reporting to managers
  - low-level reliance on historical data.
▼ *Focus*:
  - the mechanism must clearly connect income with expenditure
  - it must work within the spending cycle (e.g. the financial year)
  - the mechanism should make use of the control points characterised by the various events in the supply chain
  - there must be clear accountability.
▼ *Participation*:
  - compliance with a mutually agreed financial plan
  - active financial management
  - effective intervention techniques and tactics
  - targeting of significant variations
  - improving performance.
▼ *Change management*:
  - moving towards altered care balance
  - identifying changing patterns of spending
  - reducing turbulence and containing hostility.

# Profiles and mobility

Where a climate of change is prevalent, the danger is that the resources supporting a service may become so mobile (people leave!) that service capacity is impaired, or resources may be so stagnant that no change is possible (the estate loses its commercial value, etc.). In a development situation, demand for resources which are perceived to be more available tends to have priority, and where rationalisation of services is necessary a greater degree of mobility is required. There is therefore a need to balance flexibility against stability in resource structures.

The stability of an organisation's resource structure is illustrated in Figure 7.1, where comparisons of the distribution of resource mobility between stable and flexible resource structures are graded according to potential lifespans and availability (e.g. materials have a shorter lifespan than estate, but can usually be obtained more readily).

Increasing mobility and availability can be achieved by reducing the potential lifespan of resources through greater dependence on leasing, the employment of temporary staff, overtime, etc. However, in the rationalisation situation, a critical mobility mass may develop. Similarly, in a development

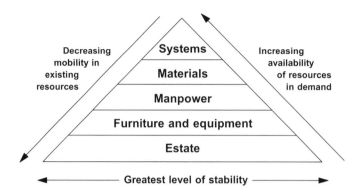

**Figure 7.1** Resources (other than finance) mobility and availability structure.

situation, where the desired resources have a long delivery lead, the capability of the business plan may be impaired.

Long resource lifespans inevitably cause increasing running and maintenance costs. It is a phenomenon that, to a lesser extent, affects other resource categories such as manpower, equipment, transport, etc. When these running costs exceed the cost of replacement (or are approaching it), the replacement option must be considered. This means that running costs must be maintained in such a way that they can be easily associated with the particular item so that a business case can be made. Frequently it is necessary to compile this case from independent research. There are two main pressures on managers to keep the lifespan of a particular resource within manageable limits:

- a desire to have mobility
- the cost of prolonging a lifespan beyond its realistic use.

This is because of the need to identify and control them adequately, and it implies that mechanisms must extend beyond the historical reporting system, so that management intervention is not simply a reaction to cost trends, but pervades every aspect of the management of the available resources.

Timing is therefore a key element in measuring resource mobility, availability and the achievement of tasks. The following limits must be established.

- *Developments*: where managers are trying to improve services, they must ensure that the resources they need can be made available within the time-frame. Thus if the delivery time, start time or lead time is greater than the time allowed in the business plan, achievement of the proposal will fail.
- *Retraction*: where there has to be a rationalisation of resources, a consequent budget reduction and redistribution of funds will be dependent on the achievement of objectives within the time-frame. Where costs are of

a continuous nature (e.g. payroll, rentals and other contractual obligations), these will continue to mount up until a suitable form of intervention is activated.

A simple budget profile can be created according to the type of budget we want to manage. A few basic steps are outlined in the checklist below.

---

**Checklist of elements and steps involved in creating a simple profile**

▼ By referring to historical patterns, calculate the amount required for regularly occurring expenditure, the basic payroll elements, the regular goods and services payments and store withdrawals, etc.

▼ Examine the list of non-recurring items, and prioritise competing demands and balance with the remainder.

▼ At this juncture, it is also worth putting aside a contingency reserve to cover exceptional and unexpected demands.

▼ Re-examine as appropriate, and approve non-recurring demands.

▼ Divide the total money available for the particular period into the appropriate category, making sure that it balances.

▼ Take the recurring budget and apportion it equally over the period according to the number of discernible segments (e.g. the yearly total weekly wages would be apportioned week by week).

▼ Keep back the non-recurring portion, adding it in only as specific expenditure occurs.

---

# Better structural arrangements

Delegation of spending authority is an important facet of any system, and some form of report and dialogue is necessary. The ability to delegate is a crucial management competence that facilitates the division of labour. It ranges from simple task sharing to specialisation in routine performance of the individual components of more complex operations. Its appropriate application is essential to successful organisational growth, but is limited by factors such as the following:

• the complexity of tasks entrusted to lower levels
• the depth relative to the organisational structure of responsibility and authority delegated
• the accountability of the delegate.

However, where budget managers appear to have maximum delegated authority and responsibility, in that they may be given both purchasing power and the ability to negotiate contracts and pay, they can still be subject to inevitable environmental pressures which are outside control.

The delegation of spending powers to lower levels of an organisation implies hierarchical recognition of greater sophistication and complexity, and the acceptance that, in reality, the rate of resource consumption is generated by staff who are neither accountants nor members of the board. However, in budgetary management it is important to truly reflect the needs of the organisation, so that the delegation process is not simply geared to the cult of already powerful managers. The decision as to where these should be allocated must always be dependent on factors which limit the range, size and scope of care levels.

Health and social care structures tend to be surprisingly flexible because they are built on a mixture of divisional rules that favour the multidisciplinary approach. Thus location – like a hospital site, for example, or a residential home or specialised unit – might form the basis of departmentism. This is illustrated in Figure 7.2.

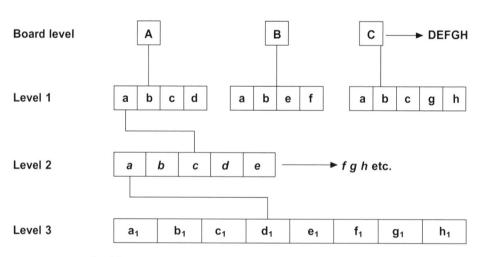

**Figure 7.2**   Flexible structure.

This model offers much more flexibility, as the manager at each level can make decisions about the whole spectrum of activity. Although the communication string would be shortened, control is exercised at various levels to ensure that this is balanced by accountability. Thus the manager has clear responsibility and authority.

# Budget viability

If departments are too large, they become difficult to control. However, if they are too small, there may be a waste of resources and it is likely that there will not be enough work to maintain a viable specialised team in practice. Budgets should be large enough to absorb reasonable fluctuations without creating a sense of crisis, but should also be reflective of the management realities.

- Maximum delegation means more budget centres but much smaller budgets.
- Selective delegated spending power result in larger budgets and fewer budget managers.
- Optimum delegation occurs when there is a regularity to budget sizes that produces the greatest flexibility.

Although health and social care organisations are seldom homogeneous in nature, it is possible to simplify the situation and calculate how a structure might evolve.

If the total value of the business within an organisation is $T$, this must be equal to the total number of departments ($n$) multiplied by the size of each share ($t$):

$$T = nt.$$

This is illustrated in Figure 7.3 below.

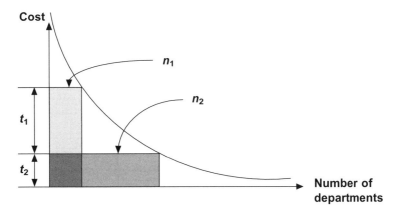

**Figure 7.3**    Cost and number of departments.

The shaded area bounded by the curve at any point will, according to the equation, always have equal values. Thus in Figure 7.3, $(t_1 * n_1) = (n_2 * t_2)$.

Where there are frequent wide spans of management to accommodate the diversity of service provision, and there are also deep structures with many levels to provide for the intensely specialised nature of some procedures, there is great potential for wastage resulting from undue overlap or from duplication of attributes. Evaluation of structure in the context of business planning seeks to identify such areas.

Apart from the departmental overlap that is necessary with regard to vertical and lateral structures, the best-known area where sharing occurs is probably the provision of administrative support to individual departments (e.g. ward clerks, receptionists, sub office staff). Another example would be where similar departments exist on one site. All organisational structures and departments need to be examined in order to determine whether there is an opportunity for rationalisation.

Figure 7.4 illustrates the process.

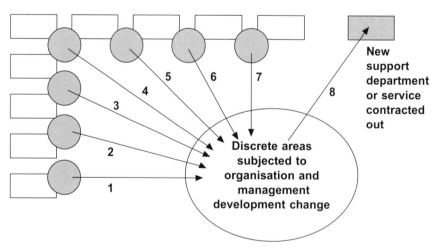

**Figure 7.4**   Potential for restructuring.

---

**The 'Do' checklist**

▼   *Do clarify relationships.* This is especially important where professional, functional or locational divisions in the organisation are already well-established practice. For example, confusion can easily arise in complex organisations where, with multidisciplinary working, individuals of equal rank may not have similar delegated authority.

▼ *Do make sure that delegation is at an appropriate organisational level.* Delegation of tasks, responsibility for whole tranches of work and/ or appropriate decision making to other levels and spheres must be carefully judged to enhance performance. There are a number of sophisticated tests which can help to assess where exactly this point should be. However, the limits are well recognised:
  – delegating too far or excessive delegation causes self-perpetuating splinters and satellites with quasi-authority
  – not delegating far enough or too little delegation results in constant referrals for ratification of minor decisions.

▼ *Do ensure that responsibility carries commensurate authority.* It is virtually impossible to delegate responsibility successfully without granting the necessary authority. If this quite common error is perpetuated in an organisation, it will lead to frustration and ultimately to failure.

▼ *Do take care that managers who have delegated powers and responsibility are aware of their accountability.* Managers at all levels are sometimes unaware of the fact that the famous axiom 'delegation is not abdication' applies to them.

▼ *As far as possible, do maintain an open system of communication.* This means that the flow of non-confidential organisational information is not restricted to chains of command, but is available on general release. Make every effort to release promptly organisational information that conforms with transparency.

---

**Tips from the front office**

▼ Arranging the transfer of powers, responsibilities and accountability, and managing the outcomes, can be costly.

▼ If there is more than one tier (e.g. in the public sector), these costs can escalate at an alarming rate.

▼ A balance has to be struck between the number and size of organisational strata and the cost incurred in simply managing them.

# Workloads and dependencies

Although dependency, as an aspect of quality, must be managed through an infrastructure that is designed both to stimulate improvement and to maintain standards, in many respects measurements are reflections on intangible benefits. It would be a useless exercise indeed to implement an expensive system that, in the long run, at one extreme end of the dependency spectrum discouraged patients or clients by intrusive questioning, or at the other end of the spectrum encouraged dependency by a mechanism of over-protection.

Whatever the advantages of the intangible beneficial weights, statements of cost and volume are as important frontline indicators of quality and dependency as they are of workload. In other words, in order to obtain the full picture, a whole range of measurement issues must be considered, but basic facts are contained in readily available statistical tables.

Cost and volume measurements represent an important relationship between patient and client volumes and resource consumption. This is usually expressed as an average cost per item (i.e. the total cost divided by the total volume). In the example of men digging a hole, it is apparent that, depending on the size of the hole and other factors, increasing the number of men and/or other resources would only improve matters up to an optimum point. Thereafter, the site would become cluttered and efficiency would be reduced.

In other words, although the total cost would be increasing, the *average* cost would fall until a point of maximum efficiency was reached, and then the *average* cost would begin to rise.

At a particular dependency level, the average cost can be calculated according to the specification for a range of workload values. As workload increases, the average cost will fall until a point of optimum efficiency is reached.

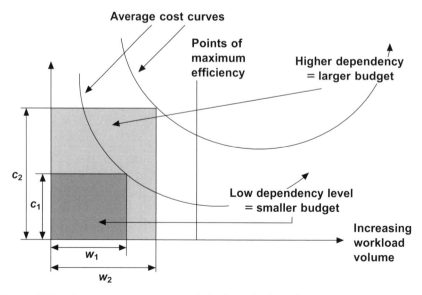

**Figure 7.5** Average cost curve and the best budget fit.

As is shown in Figure 7.5, at any particular point the total cost, or the value of the budget, is found by multiplying the workload ($w$-values) by the average agreed cost ($c$-values) for that dependency level.

Figure 7.5 also illustrates this classic connection between dependency, cost, workload and the best-fit budget.

- In the case of the low-dependency curve, the best-fit budget is $c_1 \times w_1$.
- For the higher-dependency group, the best-fit budget is $c_2 \times w_2$.

Unfortunately, managers are sometimes inclined to ignore this relationship and seek savings from existing arrangements. Where a specification is part of a contract, this must be changed in order to comply with revised funding. This does not mean that managers should cease their pursuit of more cost-effective ways of working. Moreover, where otiose resources are perceived, particularly in connection with estate, it does not follow that with a commensurate increase in staffing these can safely be brought into use without the danger of a knock-on effect further along the dependency chain, or hazards remaining undetected in the creation of unsafe practices.

Two examples can be cited here.

- Many operating theatres are not used during the evening, at night or at weekends. Theoretically, taking account of cleansing and other maintenance requirements, some of these could be brought into use with the introduction of shift systems. However, there would be accommodation and other problems elsewhere in cases where spare capacity was not so obvious (e.g. wards, etc.).
- Many community resource centres and sheltered workshops close during unsociable hours. These could be used to accommodate increases in the volume of respite care provision. However, the same kinds of arguments apply.

---

**Checklist of manageable cost components**

▼ *Elements*: the total cost of care is a mixture of two elements, namely the *fixed cost* and the *variable cost*. In perfect conditions (where there is no ageing, obsolescence, or sudden changes in care and treatment regimes) a number of phenomena occur.

▼ *Fixed costs*: these are usually thought of as the costs incurred in purchasing and/or maintaining estate and equipment. In the case of care and treatment, sometimes absolute minimum levels of staff and materials are also included. This cost will remain the same until maximum capacity is reached. After that, additional estate and equipment will be needed.

▼ *Variable costs*: these are the costs directly influenced by the volume of work undertaken, which gradually increase with increasing workload. They are usually considered to include payroll and materials.

▼ *Volumes increase*: as they do so, the variable cost increases but the fixed cost remains the same.

▼ *Average cost*: this falls to a point where maximum efficiency is achieved. This occurs even though the *total* amount is increasing. Thereafter, the average cost begins to rise because of disproportionate increases in both the fixed and variable costs.

▼ *Cost mobility*: costs are said to have cost mobility in two directions. First, there is the mobility described above, where there is movement because of increases in volume. The second type occurs during the time scale in which the cost is incurred. Thus mobility can be influenced either by the passage of time or by the volume that is handled. These two factors have important consequences when we begin to examine how costs can best be controlled.

▼ *Predictability*: although it might be reasonably expected that those costs which are described as fixed would not display any variation characteristics, in fact for a number of reasons they are subject to fluctuations. In other words, despite the fact that the total cost is constant, either the supply of the fixed-cost items may be irregular or the demand for payment may not be made in equal increments.

The problem is compounded by insatiable demands and increasing expectations of ever better management. And the climate of constant change and movement creates yet more financial difficulties.

Sometimes managers can become disheartened by an apparently permanent state of deficiency management. However, their efforts in facilitating change can be compensations in themselves. As was discussed in Chapter 4, the essential elements of their plans usually involve moving towards the appropriate balance of care provision and determining the following:

• the service core that was to be *maintained*
• *developmental* aspects and consequences required to deal with unmet need, or improvements in method or technique
• service aspects whose use or future prospects were decreasing and *rationalisation* was required.

In order to ensure that services do not become damaged at any stage in the process by immobilising resource factors that cannot cope adequately with change, there is a need to create resource structures that are flexible. In stabilising existing services, or in cases where an alteration in the balance of care is required, the quality, consumption, availability and mobility of the resources used to support these services are key factors in creating and managing the movement needed to accommodate service change and improvement.

---

### Checklist of system improvements

▼ Make compromises between maximum delegation and flexibility in order to produce a spending range that can be managed.

▼ Check for inappropriate or ineffective delegation, e.g. if there are too many management tiers, the right of veto can inexplicably impair progress.

▼ Consider the cost and benefit of enhancing potential budget managers' competences.

▼ Revise acceptability criteria.

▼ Remember that potential budget managers are usually drawn from non-financial backgrounds and may not have business acumen skills, but the fact that their departments generate significant expenditure means that unsuitable individuals must often be considered.

▼ It is important for first-time frontline managers to note that average costs vary not only due to patient/client volumes, but also because dependencies may change. For example, increased turnover rates due to shorter stays usually result in higher dependency.

▼ Clear and agreed objectives therefore have to be set together with the provision of training and expert support.

▼ Costs and benefits have to be taken into account, and if necessary the outcome of the above rules (homogeneity, size, viability, etc.) needs to be recast.

# 8

# Administration matters

Frontline staff and managers can suddenly find themselves 'in the chair' or in a position where they have to organise, co-ordinate or act as secretary to a meeting. However, no successful professional administrator performs any of these tasks without considerable preparation.

Frontline staff and first-time managers often 'manage by the seat of their pants' and stumble through the business. Usually they are unaware of the time wasting and the pitfalls they may have accidentally avoided. Hundreds (or in the case of larger units, thousands) of meetings, both formal and informal, take place during any one week. They may be connected with the care and treatment of patients or clients, or they may have a 'business' orientation.

However, regardless of scale, unless they conform to a few simple rules, they are likely to achieve little, and valuable time will be lost, only to be replaced by possible bad feeling and resentment. The simple rules are as follows.

- Meetings have to be properly convened (called or summoned).
- Notice or summons must be diligently sent to all parties who have an interest (legal entitlement, professional, etc.).
- An agenda is circulated providing information about the specific purposes or intentions of the meeting.
- A record is kept of the circumstances and decisions taken.
- Efforts are made to implement these decisions through an established communication network.
- Where consultation is required, an adequate and approved methodology is invoked.

This chapter provides guidance on all of these matters.

# The issues

Checklist of some relevant general points

▼    Do not waste time on meetings unless there is a reasonable expectation of achieving their objectives.
▼    Make sure that everyone knows well in advance what is on the agenda.
▼    An agenda should contain the following information:
  – name, date, time and place of meeting
  – apologies
  – minutes of previous meeting
  – matters arising from the minutes
  – detained reports (finance, statistics, clinical or professional matters, any reports previously commissioned, etc.)
  – correspondence
  – date of next meeting.
▼    Where small working parties are concerned, agreement by a majority, with a strong minority opposed to an idea, is not recommended.
▼    Neither an acquiescent minority nor an abstaining minority are satisfactory reflections on the strength of argument.
▼    Although it has been described as management by the lowest common denominator, try to obtain a consensus on each issue.
▼    Keep a record of what took place, when, and who was there.
▼    Confirm any agreements that are made in writing.
▼    The co-ordinator or secretary does not usually have any authority, but works by agreement of the meeting.
▼    In English, the word 'chair' is gender neutral and should not be used to describe the person who has control of the meeting's business.
▼    The word 'agenda' is the plural version of 'agendum', but it usually functions as a singular. It means a comprehensive list of matters to be discussed at a meeting.

Checklist of arrangements to be made when organising the next meeting

▼    Book the venue. Make sure that it is convenient to the majority and accessible to all.
▼    Book the audio-visual equipment and make sure that any other necessary conferencing facilities are available.

▼ Book the refreshments. Check the price and who pays.
▼ Draft the minutes or notes of the first meeting if required. Check it out!
▼ Draft any outgoing letters.
▼ Obtain an up-to-date circulation list including protocols relating to senior officers who receive details on a 'for information only' basis (e.g. professional line managers).
▼ Gather all correspondence and chase up any reports.
▼ Agree drafts, including the agenda, with the chairperson, and cover all business points.
▼ Complete the minutes, notes, agenda and outgoing correspondence.
▼ Obtain all of the necessary signatures.
▼ Distribute the minutes with any enclosures (reports, etc.) according to the list of members, etc.
▼ Accept any apologies and check the acceptability of any proposed delegate.

## On the day before the meeting

▼ Check the availability of the venue.
▼ Check that refreshments will be available at a specified time.
▼ Check the heating, air-conditioning, plugs, lights, etc.

## On the day of the meeting, allowing time for remedial action in the event of omissions

▼ Check that the doors to the venue and toilets are unlocked and accessible.
▼ Recheck the housekeeping arrangements.
▼ Set up the venue, including place settings, screens, connections, etc.
▼ Have spare copies of all documents and a supply of paper and pencils/pens available.
▼ Obtain the signature of every properly accredited member who is attending. This will be a permanent record of all those present.

---

**Tips from the front office**

▼ Focus on the business – try to be facilitating.
▼ Do not upstage or correct a senior manager – choose a private moment.
▼ Do not make enemies.

# Case study

## Sample notice of meeting and agenda

### Notice of Monthly Near-Home Management Team Meeting

The next meeting of the Near-Home Management Team will take place in the **Near-Home Facility Conference Room** at 3.00p.m. on Tuesday 12 August 2003.

### Agenda

Apologies
Minutes of previous meeting held on 8 July 2003 (attached)
Matters arising from the Minutes:

> Clerical support: Ms N Rightly to report
> Progress Report on Near-Home facility implementation

Reports:

> Financial Report presented by Mr M Luckpenny
> Statistical Information presented by Trust Information Officer
> Progress on transport

Correspondence
Any other business
Date of next meeting

# Defining and improving communications

Communications become dynamic when they rely on all of the senses. They stimulate and generate action through motivation and leadership. However, as organisations do not possess a natural charisma, communicating decisions to or seeking advice from both the internal and external environments often causes unnecessary problems.

In the external environment, health scares, inflamed passions over certain social problems, and concerns about jobs are all familiar large-scale 'negatives'. Internally, communicating with the individual patient, relative, staff member or contractor is equally important, and details such as 'who signs the letter' need attention in every organisation.

The other important aspect of communication is to achieve action – to put into practice that which:

- is the preferred option
- has been exposed to debate
- is the product of a rational decision-making process.

Much of this aspect of the communication process is systematic and is effected through the organisation's recognised arrangements. It is embedded in the standards that have already been set and agreed. It may possibly, in the case of patient and client care, be reflected in protocols that are applied consistently and without hesitation.

Operating on many levels, therefore, the facility to communicate effectively is crucial and fundamental to health and social care organisations. The development of recognisable lines and methods of communication to the satisfaction of all relevant parties is essential to the confidence of the public, staff, patients and relatives in an organisation's reputation for honesty and capability.

Figure 8.1 illustrates the process for achieving quality in communications.

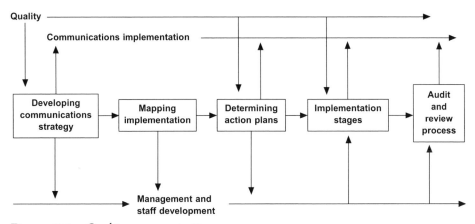

**Figure 8.1**   Quality communications.

Below is a series of short checklists of key points to remember.

---

**Checklist of administration and communication key points**

▼   Quality is implicit in the following.
  - The complex needs–wants–satisfaction chain reaction is the basic stimulus for activity in both internal and external environments.
  - Gratification of all the disparate staff and patient expectations is impossible, and there must be recognition that a degree of moderation is essential.
  - Equitable treatment, discipline and hope of an improvement are possible common denominators.
  - Fostering of the capacity for innovation and creativity in all environments is an indicator of resilient communications.

▼ Communications strategy in the human organisation
  – Strategy must be a facilitating factor in the achievement of overall objectives.
  – The structure for information dissemination should be specified, as should who speaks on what subject, approvals, etc.
  – Evolving structures tend to take on characteristics of their own, and often have a major impact on both staff performance and public confidence.
  – In sophisticated health and social care organisations there is the perception of a particular culture, as well as ethics, symbols and patient/client reputation, with which staff, the public and patients can identify.
  – Strategy should take account of the methods whereby managers are enabled to determine the degree of transparency/confidentiality that is to be applied in particular circumstances.
▼ Mapping implementation
  – The map breaks the strategy down into the expectation of improvement to be achieved within certain deadlines.
  – It sets out the specific framework to be adopted when entering a consultative process with both internal and external sources.
▼ Determining action plans
  – Action planning is the main implement for ensuring that decisions are put into practice.
  – The main component parts are broken down into manageable tasks.
  – Action plans specify deadlines within which each task must be completed.
  – They attribute specific responsibility to named officers or staff members who are then held accountable.
▼ Implementation stages
  – Defining the precision with which the communication strategy for change is to be implemented is crucial.
  – As well as the lateral process, there will also be various stands to consider (e.g. patients, clients, relatives and the public, as opposed to staff and business communications).
▼ Management and staff development
  – Staff must have adequate rewards, job satisfaction, prospects and a sense of security: they also need to know where they stand as far as organisational plans are concerned.
  – Training programmes and involvement are essential to building an effective communication network with staff.
  – This helps them feel secure and display competence and exude confidence.

- Taking the will to work, binding it into a co-operative effort and giving it direction is a vital communication characteristic.
▼ Audit and review
  - This process will follow along the lines defined in Chapter 1.
  - It will be dedicated to testing systems and structures.
  - Whether the organisation, the individual, and the individual in the organisation are consistently *doing the right thing, first time, every time* are central questions in the review and audit process.

# Case study

Action plan for the development of transport request protocols
Near-Home facility

**Strategic objective**

Development of protocols for the acceptance of transport requests for urgent and non-urgent transport services.

| Details of task | Manager/team responsible | Completion date in 2003 |
| --- | --- | --- |
| Form team from all relevant disciplines | Trust Chief Executive Officer (CEO) | August |
| Statistical survey of current level of urgent/non-urgent requests and responses to them | Information manager | 30 September |
| Segregation into patient/client types (acute, elderly, rehabilitation, etc.) | Information manager | 30 September |
| Analysis of journeys and mileage | Transport manager | First week of October |
| Costing various options | Treasurer | Second week of October |
| Consulting with interested parties | Project team leader | 31 October |
| Drafting protocols (who, when, where, how, etc.) for discussion at all levels | Team leader/team | 7 November |
| Agreeing final arrangements | CEO/trust | 14 November |
| Setting review date and criteria | CEO/trust | 14 November |

**Checklist of considerations when preparing and evaluating reports and correspondence**

▼ *Context*: make sure that the previous reference, date, title, author and audience are included. Some description and background may be necessary.

▼ *Confidentiality and transparency*: the expected level of dedication and privacy to be accorded the document should be indicated.

▼ *Complexity*: length and tedious detail are often frustrating features of reports and correspondence. Busy recipients want essential detail and the options for remedial or other action.

▼ *Format*: where considerable amounts of description and supporting data are necessary:
  – a *management summary* of salient points and recommendations can be placed at the front
  – this can be followed by a detailed *commentary*
  – finally, relevant supporting statistical, technical and cost data can be included in referenced *appendices*
  – major reports would be read from the front but prepared from the back.

▼ *Accuracy and clarity*:
  – concentrate on the facts
  – use familiar terminology with the minimum of technical terms
  – aim not to confuse or obfuscate
  – avoid the use of negatives and double negatives.

▼ *Timing and deadlines*: do not be tempted to judge a good time or a bad time to present a report. Stick to previously agreed deadlines. Leave plenty of scope both for the reader to absorb the report and for discussion.

**Tips from the front office**

▼ Remember that written communication is your chance to set out your stall and make an impression.

▼ Treat it as a personal advertisement, but do not be tempted into 'small-print trickery.' In the long run, confused customers become impatient customers.

▼ Strive to be objective.

▼ Do not make or commit to paper derogatory remarks about another person.

▼ Avoid external sensitive issues.

# Index

action plans   49, 50–1, 98
  case study   99–100
acute services, planning   51–2
administration   93–100
  case study   96
  communications   96–9
  issues   94–5
  meetings   93–100
aims
  process quality   23
  this book's   vi–vii
amalgamation, planning   47
audit
  planning   44
  project management   8, 11

beneficiaries, this book's   vii
budgets   6
  checklist   83, 86–7
  communication characteristics   80–1
  cost components   89–90
  dependencies   87–91
  issues   79–81
  management systems   79–91
  mobility   81–3
  planning   45
  profiles   81–3
  restructuring   85–7
  structural arrangements   83–4
  system improvements   91
  viability   85–7
  workloads   87–91
  see also resources
bureaucracy, basic   3–4

case studies
  action plans   99–100
  administration   96
  gifts   19–21
  meetings   96

payroll   67
planning   51–2
readmission   12–13
rehabilitation   12–13
resources   77
security   36
staff   67
cash   25–36
  checklist   26–8
  issues   26–8
  patient/client monies   29–30
  see also budgets; fund raising; money
catchment area, planning   46
change, influencing factors   38–9
commissioning equipment, supply chain   60
communications
  administration   96–9
  defining   96–9
  improving   96–9
competence, culture of   vii–viii, 1–13,
     63–5
confusion, planning   46
considerations see gifts
consultation process, project management
     10
contingency management, supply chain
     62–3
correspondence, checklist   100
costs see budgets
culture of competence   vii–viii, 1–13
  payroll   63–5

data sources, project management   9–10
delivery, supply chain   60
dependencies, budgets   87–91

ethical pressures, planning   45
exchange dilemma, resources   74–5
expenditure   4, 6
  see also budgets; resources

financial periods, prioritising during   74–6
frontline staff
    administration   93–100
    defined   1
    supply chain   54–6
fund raising   30–4
    checklist   31–4
    steering groups   31–2
funding gaps, bridging   76
funding sources   76

gifts   15–23
    acceptability criteria   17–19
    acceptable material   22
    agreement   17–18
    appropriateness   18
    case study   19–21
    co-ordination   22
    communication   22
    communication gap   18–19
    costs   18
    defined   16
    external influences   21
    guiding protocol principles   21
    harmony   18
    internal constraints   21
    key issues   16–17
    management structure   18
    practical steps   22–3
    review   22
    seven Ps   23
    utility   17–18

hospitality see gifts

inaccessibility, planning   46
income   3–4
internal constraints, gifts   21
internal developments, resources   70
internal environment, resources   71–2
internal/external environments, planning
    39–41
internal procedures, security   35

key stages, project management   9–12

legal pressures, planning   45
liability considerations, planning   45
loss, supply chain   57–60

management systems, budgets   79–91
management tips, project management
    11–12
meetings
    administration   93–100
    case study   96
    checklist   94–5
    money   4
mobility, budgets   81–3
money
    meetings   4
    organisation   4
    planning   4
    resources bidding   4
    see also budgets; cash; expenditure;
        income; purchasing
moral pressures, planning   45
morale, supply chain   63–5

ombudsman, planning   44–5
operational plans   49
opportunities, planning   45–6
organisation, money   4

patient/client monies, money management
    29–30
payment, supply chain   60
payroll
    accuracy   65–7
    case study   67
    culture of competence   63–5
    protocols   66–7
    supply chain   63–7
pilfering   28–9
planning
    action plans   49, 50–1, 98, 99–100
    activation   50
    amalgamation   47
    analysis   41–7
    audit   44
    budgets   45
    case study   51–2
    catchment area   46
    change, influencing factors   38–9
    checklist   39–40
    confusion   46
    current position   47
    environments   39–41
    essentials   37–52

ethical pressures   45
features, fundamental   39–40
historical position   47–8
inaccessibility   46
information   41–7
internal/external environments   39–41
issues   37–9
legal pressures   45
liability considerations   45
money   4
moral pressures   45
ombudsman   44–5
operational plans   49
opportunities   45–6
pressure groups   45
processes   38
professional inspection   44
project management   7
quality initiatives   48
resources   48
restructuring   46
retraction models   46–7
roll-out plans   49, 50–1
security   45
sense of direction   40–1
shaping the plan   47–51
staff vacancies   47
strengths   41–3
SWOT analysis   41–7
threats   46–7
weaknesses   43–5
workloads   48
pressure groups, planning   45
prioritising resources   73–6
problem areas, project management   10
process failure   v–vi
process quality
   aims   2–3
   benefits checklist   2
   central theme   2–3
professional inspection, planning   44
project management   7–8
   definitions   7–8
   terminology   7–8
purchasing, supply chain   57–8, 62

quality assurance   8
   communications   96–9
   supply chain   61–2

quality initiatives, planning   48
quotation procedures, supply chain   58

readmission, case study   12–13
receipts   6
recommendations, project management   10
rehabilitation
   case study   12–13
   planning   52
reports, checklist   100
requirements, supply chain   57
resources
   additional, bidding for   69–77
   case study   77
   checklist   5–6
   condition of   72
   essential   5–6
   exchange dilemma   74–5
   financial criteria   70–1
   funding gaps, bridging   76
   funding sources   76
   implications   10
   internal developments   70
   internal environment   71–2
   issues   69–71
   listing demands   71–2
   planning   48
   prioritising   73–6
   tendering procedures   58
   see also budgets; expenditure; supply chain
resources bidding, money   4
respite care, case study   12–13
restructuring
   budgets   85–7
   planning   46
retraction models, planning   46–7
review
   gifts   22
   project management   8, 11
   supply chain   62–3
robbery   28–9
roll-out plans   49, 50–1

samples testing, supply chain   59
security   25–36
   case study   36
   improvements   34–6
   internal procedures   35
   issues   26–8

security (*continued*)
   organisation 34–5
   planning 45, 52
   response plan 35–6
   strategy 34–6
   systems 35
selection, supply chain 58
sense of direction, planning 40–1
sourcing, supply chain 58
staff
   case study 67
   frontline 1, 54–6, 93–100
   mobility 81–3
   morale 63–5
   payroll 63–7
   vacancies 47
stagnation, case study 12–13
standardisation, supply chain 58
stealing 28–9
stock items, supply chain 59
strengths, planning 41–3
structure, this book's viii–ix
supply chain
   checklist 54, 57–60
   contingency management 62–3
   dos and don'ts 61–2
   frontline staff 54–6
   influencing 53–67

   issues 53–6
   loss 57–60
   morale 63–5
   payroll 63–7
   purchasing 57–8, 62
   quality assurance 61–2
   review 62–3
   summary chart 56
   top tips 55–62
   waste 57–60
   *see also* resources
SWOT analysis, planning 41–7

tendering procedures
   supply chain 58
   *see also* resources
threats 28–9
   planning 46–7
training programmes, project
     management 11
transport services, planning 51

waste, supply chain 57–60
weaknesses, planning 43–5
workloads
   budgets 87–91
   planning 48